Beating Heart Disease: Your Guide to a Healthier You

Anton

TABLE OF CONTENTS

CHAPTER I: Introduction

1.1 Cardiovascular Diseases

Cardiovascular diseases (CVDs) are disorders that afflict the heart and blood vessels. CVD are a leading cause of morbidity and mortality globally in both men and women[1]. In the United States alone, it's estimated that one person succumbs to CVD every 33 seconds[1,2]. In the year 2021, CVD caused 20.5 million mortalities worldwide, accounting for roughly one-third of all global fatalities. In the USA, annually, 697,000 lives are lost to CVD and about 121.5 million adults suffer from quality of life issues and require medical management with one or more manifestations of CVD[3]. The economic burden of this disease is staggering, with direct and indirect costs totaling around $239.9 billion annually[2].

Manifestations of CVD include coronary heart disease (CHD), stroke, hypertension, congestive heart failure, peripheral artery disease, rheumatic heart disease, deep vein thrombosis, atherosclerosis, and aneurysms. The multifactorial nature of CVDs can be attributed to multiple modifiable or manageable risk factors such as diet, obesity, smoking, stress, and alcohol consumption. Unmodifiable risk factors include age, heredity, gender, and more[4]. Treatment for CVD varies, encompassing lifestyle adjustments, medication, surgical procedures, and device implantation. Surgical interventions become necessary when passive management proves ineffective. Nevertheless, standard treatments come with inherent risks, including allergic reactions, bleeding (especially with blood thinners), and potential liver and kidney side effects with medication-based treatment. Surgery and device implantation may lead to complications such as infection, adverse reactions to anesthesia, blood clots, hyperplasia, severe inflammation due to biocompatibility issues, and endoleaks, often signaling to device failure. Given the limitations and risks associated with current treatment strategies, there is a pressing need for alternative approaches that address these shortcomings and enhance their efficacy in reducing CVD mortality rates. Among the spectrum of cardiovascular diseases, special attention must be directed towards aortic aneurysms, particularly AAAs, due to their substantial impact on global health, high mortality rates, and the lack of non-surgical treatment approaches to reverse their pathophysiology.

1.2   Abdominal Aortic Aneurysms

AAAs are localized, naturally irreversible expansions of the abdominal aorta wall that typically occur in the infrarenal part (between renal arteries and aortic bifurcation) of the aorta. These aneurysms have consistently ranked as the 10th to 15th leading cause of death, primarily affecting older males over the past decades, and they carry a daunting 90% mortality rate upon rupture[5,6]. AAAs undergo slow, progressive growth over several years, often culminating in rupture, which usually proves fatal. They predominantly afflict elderly males (~4-9%), with a lower prevalence among females (1-3%), and their incidence notably increases in individuals over 60 years of age[7,8]. There is a worldwide increment in the incidence of AAAs, ranging from 4.2% to 11% per year[9]. Age, male sex, smoking, genetic predisposition, and high total cholesterol are the known risk factors which contribute to development and progression of AAAs. Risky open surgery or EVAR remains the primary options for addressing larger and more severe AAAs, and these surgical approaches account for a total of ~$10 billion in healthcare expenditure each year in the USA alone. However, there are presently no active treatments available for small AAAs that exhibit slow and gradual growth, often progressing to a dangerous pre-rupture stage over several years. Despite some evidence of clinical effectiveness, medications and other therapies have failed to reverse AAA pahophysiology[10]. Given these limitations in AAA treatment, there is a compelling need for alternative approaches that focus on slowing, halting, or potentially reversing AAA pathophysiology, with a strong emphasis on regenerative repair of the AAA wall.

The underlying pathophysiological cause of AAA formation is the chronic enzymatic breakdown of the structural extracellular matrix (ECM), mostly collagen and elastic fibers of the aorta wall, by matrix metalloproteases (MMPs), following an initial injury stimulus. Collagen provides strength and resistance to vessel bursting, and elastic fibers allow the vessel to stretch and recoil (elasticity) to accommodate blood flow and maintain blood pressure. However, the etiology of AAAs is highly multifactorial, additionally involving the infiltration of leucocytes and production of ranges of pro-inflammatory cytokines and proteases, destruction of vascular smooth muscle cell (VSMC), phenotypic modulation of VSMCs between contractile and synthetic phenotypes, endothelial dysfunction and loss of nitric oxide (NO) signaling [11,12]. Persistence cumulation of these inflammatory processes in the ECM milieu, importantly the concomitant breakdown of the matured cross-linked elastic matrix, which is a critical determinant of abnormal vessel expansions, make the aorta vulnerable to forces generated by the internal pressure leading to loss of aortal wall elasticity, weakening, and fatal stress-induced rupture of the aorta wall.

1.3   Study Rationale

The persistent adverse microstructural changes in elastin and collagen fiber architecture and content owed to overexpressed proteases, along with the deficient and impaired natural processes for regenerative repair of elastic matrix in adult and diseased vascular tissues currently impede therapeutic reversal of AAA pathophysiology. Poor elastic matrix neoassembly and repair are challenged by the intrinsically deficient synthesis of elastin precursors (tropoelastin), by adult and more so, diseased vascular cells. These cells are also impaired in their ability to replicate the biocomplexity of elastic fiber assembly, which primarily occurs during the post-neonatal phase[13]. This deficiency represents a critical "missing link" within natural tissue remodeling responses to injury. Consequently, there is a critical need for matrix regenerative therapies capable of addressing these shortcomings. Such therapies would hold the potential to significantly impact the restoration of the elastic matrix in AAAs by fostering the regenerative repair process, thus offering a promising avenue for effective intervention in this intricate and challenging condition.

Recent research highlights NO, a potent vasodilator, capable of downregulating MMPs and enhancing the expression of tissue inhibitors of MMPs (TIMPs)[14]. However, in the context of inflammatory AAAs, existing literature suggests that mitogen-activated protein kinases (MAPKs), including c-Jun N-terminal kinase (JNK) and extracellular-signal-regulated kinase (ERK), are upregulated[15,16]. This leads to downstream cytokine-induced SMC apoptosis and upregulation of elastases such as cathepsin K[17,18]. In prior work conducted by the Ramamurthi group, MAPK inhibition was found to downregulate elastolytic MMPs, stimulate elastin protein synthesis, and cross-linked elastic fiber formation by aneurysmal SMCs through increases in transforming growth factor β1 (TGF-β1), a cytokine which has been identified as pro-elastogenic[13,19,20]. Thus, there is compelling rationale and motivation to explore the pro-elastogenic and anti-MMP effects of select NO donor drugs, as a function of exogenous dose. Others have also shown endogenous NO to suppress JNK activation inhibit apoptosis, and inhibit robust SMC proliferation[21,22]. Thus, NO delivery drugs could potentially provide multimodal benefits to restoring elastic matrix homeostasis in the AAA wall via the mechanism of MAPK inhibition.

Oral prophylaxis of NO donor drugs for AAA treatment faces considerable limitations, primarily due to the short half-life of NO (2-6s), adverse side effects, and most importantly uncertain drug pharmacokinetics in the gut which results in the loss of drug integrity and efficacy[23,24]. Synthetic polymer-based nanoparticles (NPs) have emerged as promising solutions for tissue-localized and controlled drug delivery. They can potentially improve the local efficacy of the drug and mitigate the extensive loss of the drugs during the adsorption process through the gut[24,25]. Notably, poly(ethylene glycol) (PEG)- poly(lactic-co-glycolic acid (PLGA) based NPs have gained traction for cardiovascular theranostic applications (such as in AAAs). Our lab has previously developed a first-generation design of PEG-PLGA NPs that are especially surface-functionalized to provide drug-independent elastic matrix regenerative stimuli[26,27]. However, the use of these polymeric NPs for therapeutic applications is limited by several disadvantages including residual organic solvents, cytotoxicity of the degraded products, poor tissue penetration, incomplete drug release or drug leakage, and instability in their membrane fluidity[28]. On the other hand, liposomes or lipid nanoparticles (LNPs), phospholipid vesicles, fabricated using natural phospholipids overcome such disadvantages and based on previously documented findings may be beneficial to stabilize therapeutic compounds, increase cellular and tissue uptake, enhance permeability and retention (EPR), minimize cytotoxicity, stabilize membrane fluidity and prevent drug leakage[29]. Moreover, LNPs boast excellent biocompatibility making them ideal for diverse biomedical applications. On another front, biodegradable polycaprolactone (PCL) finds application in tissue engineering scaffolds due to its mechanical robustness, chemical versatility, and biocompatibility with tissues[30,31]. There is thus significant motivation to investigate LNP-mediated delivery of a NO donor drug and the feasibility of using PCL grafts/meshes as a platform to present the LNPs in vivo towards therapeutically effecting on site AAA wall repair.

1.4   Study Objective, Hypothesis, and Specific Aims

In the context of the discussion in section 1.3 above, the **primary objective** of this study was to investigate the impact of delivering sodium nitroprusside (SNP), a clinically widely adopted NO donor drug, on the regeneration of the elastic matrix in a matrix-compromised vascular tissue milieu. The broad **hypothesis** tested in this work was that SNP suppresses MAPK expression in aneurysmal human aortal SMCs (aHASMCs) as a function of dose, and this evokes outcomes of enhanced elastic fiber assembly and suppressed proteolytic activity, to collectively restore elastic matrix homeostasis and thus alleviate AAA pathophysiology. The **specific activities** pursued in this project were to a) assess the *in-vitro* regenerative potential of SNP, a widely clinically used NO donor drug in human aneurysmal SMCs, and b) explore the utility of a novel SNP delivery system comprised of an LNP-charged PCL graft (LCG) to investigate its matrix restorative benefits to cellular elastic matrix regenerative repair towards *in-vivo* deployment to regress AAA matrix pathophysiology. The LCG harnesses biotin-neutravidin-biotin bonding to conjugate SNP-encapsulated biotinylated LNPs (SNP-bLNPs) to the biotinylated PCL (bPCL) scaffold. We thus performed *in-vitro* and *ex-vivo* assessment of the LCG for matrix restoration by aneurysmal SMCs.

1.5   Specific Aims (SAs)

SA1. Investigate the SNP dose effects and the underlying mechanisms on elastic matrix neoassembly and anti-proteolytic effects in a cytokine injury culture model of aHASMCs.

SA2. Characterize bPCL grafts charged with SNP-bLNPs (LCGs) as an SNP delivery system and demonstrate elastic matrix regenerative benefits in aHASMC cultures.

SA3. Generate evidence of the therapeutic efficacy of LCGs in an *ex-vivo* proteolytic injury vascular model.

1.6   Study Significance and Innovation

AAA treatment options are severely limited, with larger pre-rupture AAAs primarily requiring risky surgical procedures associated with numerous perioperative, intraoperative, and postoperative risks. Furthermore, smaller AAAs receive inadequate treatment due to the absence of effective therapies capable of halting their progression during their extended years-long growth phase. Despite numerous drugs in the development pipelined discussed further in Chapter 2 section 2.3.3, there is no convincing evidence of their clinical benefit of restoring healthy aortal ECM and arresting AAA growth [10,32]. This, therefore, justifies the dire need for regenerative therapy that can slow or stop AAAs during their years-long growth phase. This project sought to establish the feasibility of a new approach for AAA wall repair based on periodic treatment with repurposed SNP drug delivered with LCGs prepared by conjugating SNP encapsulating bLNPs. The bLNPs are designed to actively provide localized, predictable, and sustained drug release, provide synergy to pro-matrix regenerative effects of the loaded drug, SNP, for long-term anti-MMP & pro-elastogenic effects thereby regressing AAA growth. By providing the opportunity to treat an AAA early, well before it reaches a rupture stage, this approach can potentially provide a viable alternative to risky surgery, reduce need for emergency surgery associated with AAA rupture, and reduce treatment costs. As an adjuvant to EVAR, SNP-bLNP therapy could also improve long-term prognosis by arresting continued expansion of the stented proximal aortic neck, a cause of graft failure[33]. Differently, by calibrating potency of MAPK inhibition to quantitative and qualitative metrices of elastic matrix assembly, we can repurpose our SNP- bLNPs to counter the challenge of poor elastic matrix generation within tissue engineered blood vessels for human use.

1.7   Scientific Innovation

The success of our matrix regenerative approach could revolutionize AAA treatment, offering a groundbreaking therapy to slow or even halt AAA growth. Repurposing a well-known vasodilator drug SNP as a catalyst to stimulate elastic matrix regeneration represents an innovative strategy. By targeting SNP-mediated MAPK inhibition, we can potentially unlock a multi-faceted cascade of downstream effects, including MMP inhibition and the stimulation of elastin synthesis and crosslinking. MAPK inhibition thus mechanistically novel in the context of both elastic matrix regeneration and also AAA treatment. This approach is expected to allow us to fine-tune elastic fiber assembly for customized matrix regenerative outcomes (e.g., modulate elastin crosslinking levels or elastic fiber size) through graded suppression of MAPKs.

Our cationic LNPs are designed to provide constant elastic matrix regenerative stimuli to aHASMCs (*in-vitro*) and while, the periadventitially implanted LCGs on the *ex-vivo* porcine carotid artery recellularized with aHASMCs, holds the potential to stimulate and engage the vascular SMCs to reprogram matrix assembly and crosslinking.

The LNPs **(Figure 1),** formulated using naturally derived phospholipids, notably 1,2-dioleoyl-3-trimethylammonium propane (DOTAP), dioleoylphosphatidylethanolamine **(DOPE)**, and cholesterol, exhibit biological compatibility, and feeble immunogenicity due to their mixed lipid chains. DOTAP confers a positive (cationic) surface charge to the LNPs, DOPE influences membrane fluidity and elasticity to promote fusion with the cells, whereas cholesterol increases the stability of the LNPs[34]. The cationic surface charge provided by DOTAP facilitates liposomal binding to the negatively charged cell membranes, potentially leading to augmentation in the drug bioavailability. PEGylation of the surface of the LNPs helps to reduce the cytotoxicity of LNPs, reduce LNP aggregation in circulation and improve circulation times by imparting the stealth properties[35]. Further enhancing the target specificity, biotin molecule guides biotinylated LNPs to bind to biotinylated-PCL graft **(Figure 1)** facilitated by covalent attachment to neutravidin, creating a precise LCG system. Additionally, the LCG could also provide mechanical reinforcement to the arteries if implanted in an *in-vivo* model. Our approach thus has the potential to create a new AAA treatment paradigm based on in situ matrix regenerative repair.

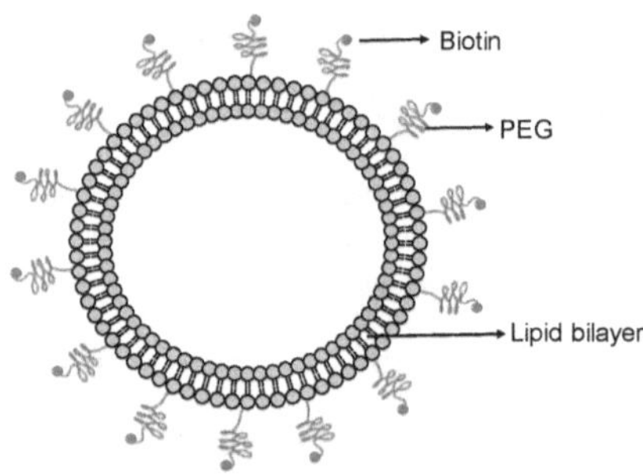

Figure 1: Schematic of biotinylated lipid nanoparticles (bLNP). The diagram showcases a lipid bilayer characterized by mol% ratios of DOTAP:DOPE:Cholesterol in 0.5:0.5:0.5. Notably, the composition includes 40 mol% of PEG-Biotin, enhancing the surface properties for potential applications in localized drug delivery. Prepared using ChemDraw

1.8   Organization of book

This book has been divided into 6 chapters. Chapter I provides the general introduction to the problem statement, motivation, and clinical significance of this study, and identifies the broad objective, hypothesis, and specific aims.

Chapter II provides a comprehensive literature review. This chapter discusses vascular anatomy and physiology, with a focus on the abdominal aorta, provides a primer on vascular wall components – cells and the extracellular matrix, and discusses vascular biology in health and disease. The chapter also provides detailed information on manifestations of vascular disorders with a focus on pathophysiology of AAAs, treatment approaches and their challenges and emerging methods for minimally invasive treatments. The chapter then provides background on the approaches and challenges to regenerative repair of the aorta wall and current and emerging state of art in terms of drug delivery for vascular regenerative outcomes.

Chapter III details the assessment of the stimulatory effects of SNP on elastic matrix neoassembly in a cytokine injury model of cultured aHASMCs and anti-proteolytic benefits. We have identified the safe and functionally beneficial SNP doses and the key intracellular mechanisms underlying their pro-regenerative effects.

Chapter IV addresses the numerous challenges associated with conventional oral drug delivery. The study detailed in this chapter explores LCGs for SNP delivery. The chapter provides information on the design, development, characterization of biotinylated LNPs, assessments of LNP stability, SNP encapsulation and encapsulation efficiency, bLNP conjugation to the bPCL graft for the formation of LCGs, their cytocompatibility with aHASMCs, and aHASMCs gene and protein expression responses to SNP released from LCGs. This chapter also provides a limited-scope proof-of-concept study that demonstrates the feasibility of LCG-stimulated elastic matrix regeneration by aHASMCs in an *ex-vivo* simulated, matrix-disrupted 3D milieu. In this chapter, we demonstrate that the LCGs offer the promise of sustained release of SNP at levels that facilitate elastic matrix neoassembly and anti-proteolytic effects in a cytokine injury in vitro aHASMC culture model —a pivotal step in the quest to combat small AAA.

Chapter VI summarizes the key findings of this book research, identifies limitations and future directions.

CHAPTER II: Background

2.1   The Arterial System

2.1.1   The Heart: Regulator of Blood Circulation

The heart, blood and the blood vessels make up the cardiovascular (or circulatory) system[36]. The heart is a highly muscular, highly automated pumping device that pumps blood around the body as it contracts. The contraction (beats) of the heart is the fundamental physiological function generated by the specialized population of cardiac cells in periodical, never-ending and fatigueless electrical oscillations. Central to its role, the heart (**Figure 2**) continuously pumps blood in and out of the heart which is then transported in and away by the networks of blood vessels (veins, arteries, and capillaries)[36]. The

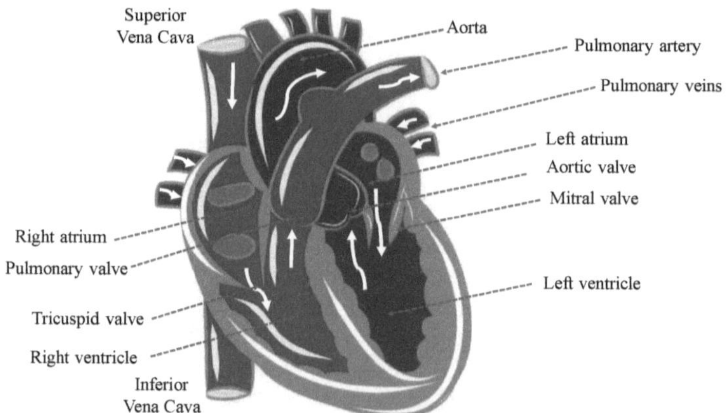

Figure 2: Anatomy of the human heart. Blood flows through the chambers and heart valves following the direction shown by the arrows. This figure was generated using images modified from Servier Medical Art, licensed under a Creative Commons Attribution 3.0 license.

transport of the blood occurs via a controlled contraction of the blood vessels that eventually offers oxygen, nutrients, and other essential material exchange to and from tissues or organs for survival. Since survival is dependent on the circulation of the blood, the cardiovascular system makes its appearance in the developing embryo as early as 4 weeks following fertilization and reaches a functional state before any other organs[37]. The cardiovascular system is vital to maintaining homeostasis; a stable, relatively constant internal environment of the body.

2.1.2   Overview of the Arterial System

Blood circulation is a one-way process that carries blood from the heart to distal tissues or back from all parts of the body to the heart. Arteries, veins, and capillaries are the primary components of the circulatory networks. Arteries play a crucial role in carrying oxygenated blood away from the heart and distributing it to various tissues. Along the way, they branch out into arterioles, leading to the smallest blood vessels known as capillaries. Capillaries possess thin vessel walls, enabling them to facilitate the exchange of respiratory gases and nutrients with specific cells. The aorta is the largest artery that originates from the left ventricle of the heart and goes all the way down to the L4 vertebral body where it bifurcates into the left and right common iliac arteries. Conversely, veins undertake the responsibility of carrying blood from the tissues back toward the heart. Lastly, capillaries, with their delicate structure, serve as the tiniest blood vessels, enabling the vital exchange of oxygen, nutrients, carbon dioxide, and waste products between the bloodstream and surrounding tissues. Together, these interconnected components form an intricate network that ensures the efficient circulation and transport of blood throughout the body.

2.1.3 Structure and Physiology of the Arterial System

Arteries, the resilient and dynamic blood vessels, consist of three intricate layers known as the intima, media, and adventitia (**Figure 3**). As they extend from the heart, arteries progressively decrease in size, with the aorta reigning as the largest artery, with a diameter of ~25 mm, while arterioles represent the smallest arteries, measuring roughly 0.3 mm. The proportions of these layers within the arterial structure vary, adapting to the size and specific functions of the arteries[38].

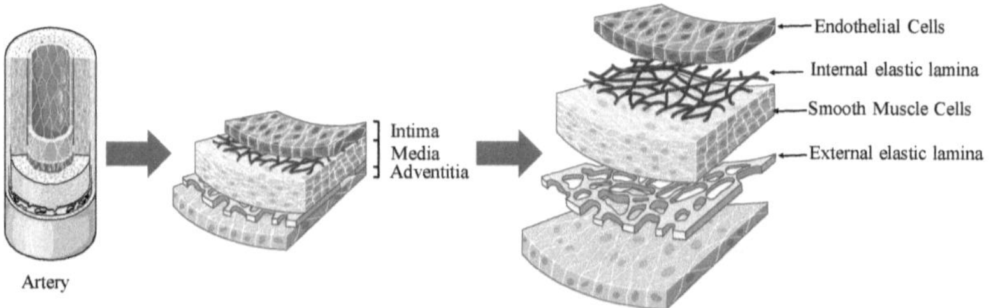

Figure 3: General structural features of arteries showing 3 distinct hierarchical layers. This figure was generated using images modified from Servier Medical Art, licensed under a Creative Commons Attribution 3.0 license.

The tunica intima serves as the innermost barrier of the vessel wall in contact with circulating blood and comprises a monolayer of endothelial cells resting upon a basal lamina that is rich in elastic fibers, collagen, and laminin. Occupying the middle layer, the tunica media, is a complex amalgamation housing VSMCs embedded within an extracellular matrix (ECM) comprised of both structural matrix components such as collagens and elastic fibers, and other ECM components such as proteoglycans and glycoproteins. External to the tunica media is the tunica adventitia layer which provides structural support and burst strength to the vessel wall. This adventitial layer consists of randomly arranged collagen fibers, dispersed fibroblasts, and a sparse population of elastic

fibers[39]. These distinct layers of the artery wall control blood pressure and enable vessel

stretch and recoil actions. These vital functions of arteries primarily rely upon the

orchestrated interplay between VSMCs and the ECM, governed by various intricate

processes and transduction pathways. Any changes in the mechanical forces or properties

may cause aberrant changes in the physiological condition leading to chronic arterial

remodeling and dysfunction.

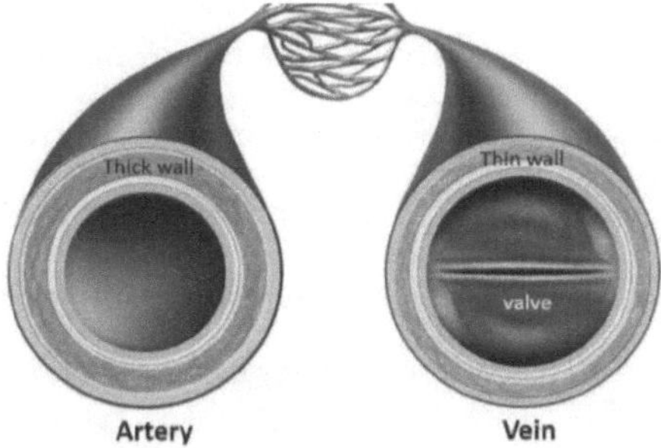

Figure 4: Figure showing anatomical differences between arteries and veins,
emphasizing differences in wall thickness, luminal diameter, and the overall
architecture[40]

Arteries differ from veins in their primary function within the circulatory system.

Arteries transport blood away from the heart to various tissues and organs, while veins

carry blood from the tissues back to the heart[36]. In terms of structural differences, veins

possess three similar layers as arteries, but they tend to have fewer VSMCs and less amount

of connective tissue within the medial layer, resulting in thinner walls **(Figure 4)** [41]. This

distinction is due to the lower pressure and more consistent blood flow in veins compared

to arteries. Arteries experience significant pressure fluctuations with each heartbeat

18

(systole and diastole), which necessitates thicker, more robust walls. In contrast, the thinner walls of veins allow them to accommodate larger blood volumes than arteries can hold at any given time[41].

2.2   Aorta: The Major Artery

2.2.1   Anatomy

The aorta is a muscular artery that carries blood coursing through the body from the heart to the farthest reaches of the limbs **(Figure 5)**. It exits the left ventricle, a powerful chamber that pumps blood out into the aorta. [42,43]. It is responsible for delivering oxygen-rich blood from the heart to every part of the body. It originates from the left ventricle, rising upward into the chest to form an arch-like structure before extending downward and branching into the iliac arteries. The key sections of the aorta are further explained below.

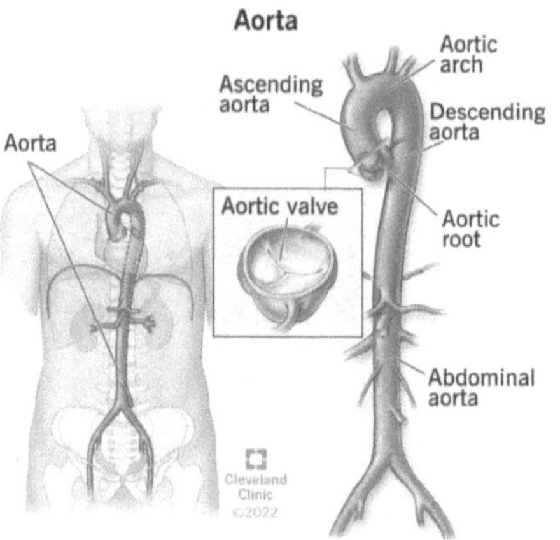

Figure 5: Diagram of aorta showing its segments, and branches [42]

2.2.1.1 Aortic Root

The aortic root is the segment of the aorta that connects to the heart and encompasses the aortic valve. The aortic valve regulates the flow of blood from the heart and prevents the regurgitation of the blood back to the ventricles. Both the right and left coronary arteries originate from the aortic root, supplying oxygen-rich blood to the heart muscles. Just like all other tissues, the heart muscle requires oxygen-rich blood to function properly.

2.2.1.2 Ascending Aorta

The ascending aorta starts right after the aortic valves in the aortic root and goes up to the aortic arch[42,43,43].

2.2.1.3 Aortic Arch

The aortic arch is shaped like an arch and connects the ascending aorta to the descending aorta. It's like a bend in the aortic root. The aortic arch gives rise to three major arteries: the brachiocephalic artery (which supplies blood to the right side of the brain and arm), the left carotid artery (which supplies blood to the left side of the brain), and the left subclavian artery (which supplies blood to the left arm)[42].

2.2.1.4 Descending aorta

The descending aorta travels down from the aortic arch through the chest and splits into the thoracic aorta and the abdominal aorta. The thoracic aorta extends from the aortic arch to just before the diaphragm. It carries blood to the chest wall and the spinal cord[43].

2.2.1.5 Abdominal Aorta

The abdominal aorta runs from the diaphragm down to just above the pelvis. It then divides into the iliac arteries, which supply blood to the legs and pelvis. Besides these main arteries, the abdominal aorta also branches into the celiac artery (which supplies blood to the stomach, liver, and pancreas), the superior mesenteric artery (which supplies the small intestine), the inferior mesenteric artery (which supplies the large intestine), and the renal arteries (which supply the kidneys, abdominal wall, and spinal cord)[43].

2.2.2 Histology

Like other arteries, the aorta is comprised of three distinct layers: the tunica intima, tunica media, and tunica adventitia (**Figure 6**) [44]. These layers work together to ensure the aorta's structural integrity and its functional capacity.

2.2.2.1 Tunica Intima

The innermost layer of the aorta's wall, the tunica intima, faces the flowing blood. It's made up of a single layer of squamous endothelial cells resting on a thin layer of connective tissue[45]. This layer helps prevent blood clots and keeps the blood moving smoothly, which is also controlled by the vessel's contracting and relaxing. Endothelial cells in this layer are the main source of NO, which controls various physiological processes such as platelet activation and aggregation, thrombus formation, vascular tone etc.[46]. The tunica intima is separated from the tunica media, the middle layer of the aorta's wall, by a part called the internal elastic lamella (IEL) or elastica interna (**Figure 6** and **Figure 7**). The tunica intima and tunica media possess elastic properties that contribute to the efficient flow of blood.

2.2.2.2   Tunica Media

The tunica media is a complex structure consisting of concentric elastic lamellae interspersed with VSMCs. The thickness of the media layer is generally proportionate to the vessel's diameter and is most pronounced in the aorta compared to other smaller arteries and veins. Comparatively, the media in veins is thinner than that found in arteries. Within this layer, VSMCs play a crucial role in the synthesis of elastin molecules, which are subsequently integrated into the elastic fibers[47,48].. These elastic fibers are instrumental in providing compliance to the arterial wall, ensuring the equilibrium of hemodynamic forces during frequent systole and diastole.

VSMCs exhibit a unique capacity to adapt their phenotypes in response to various microenvironmental factors and signals of a biochemical and biomechanical nature[49]. Moreover, they facilitate the transmission of signals to the extracellular matrix (ECM) through cell surface receptors, thereby establishing a connection between the external environment and the cytoskeleton[50]. Additionally, upon triggered by injury or certain stress activated injury stimulus, inflammatory cells such as macrophages and neutrophils infiltrate to the medial layer and activating pathways (e.g. Mitogen activated-protein kinase (MAPK) pathways) within the VSMCs[44]. This interaction leads to the activation of transcription and translation processes. The ECM that envelops VSMCs has the additional function of sequestering and releasing bioactive molecules that further influence the modulation of VSMC phenotypes[47].

2.2.2.3 Tunica Adventitia

The tunica adventitia is separated from tunica media with wavy external elastic lamina or elastica externa. External elastic lamina are usually not seen in smaller arteries and veins[51]. Tunica Adventitia constitutes the outermost layer of the aortic wall, primarily composed of collagenous extracellular matrix, fibroblasts[47]. This layer is notably rich in collagen, imparting greater tensile strength compared to the other aortic layers[52]. Moreover, the adventitia houses nerve supply and vasa vasorum **(Figure 7)**, which serve to provide essential nutrients to the aortic wall. Its primary function is to safeguard the vessel from excessive expansion and potential rupture when exposed to the high blood pressure within [53].

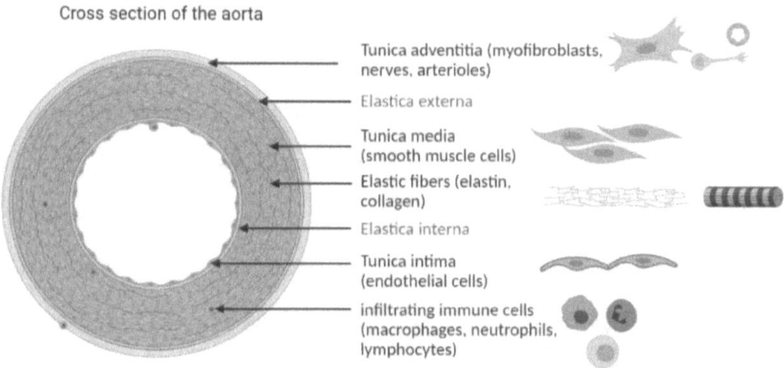

Figure 6: Cross section and composition of the aorta delineating its three distinct layers: The tunica intima, comprising an endothelial lining; the tunica media, characterized by a high concentration of elastic matrix (elastin and collagen) and multiple layers of smooth muscle cells (SMCs); and the tunica adventitia, composed of fibroblasts, nerves, and vasavasorum [44]

2.2.3   Different Cell Types and Extracellular Matrix Components in the Vessel Wall

2.2.3.1   Vascular Cells and Their Role in Remodeling

The aorta features a solitary layer of endothelial cells forming the tunica intima similar to other arteries. Directly beneath this endothelial lining **(Figure 7)** and under the internal elastic lamella (IEL), within the medial layer, there are 10-15 layers of VSMCs [54]. These VSMCs primarily serve to regulate and maintain the balance in the blood conduit process, thereby managing vessel tone, blood pressure, and blood flow. Additionally, they play a crucial role in the synthesis and remodeling of extracellular matrix components, actively contributing to the maintenance of vascular homeostasis through controlled contraction and relaxation.

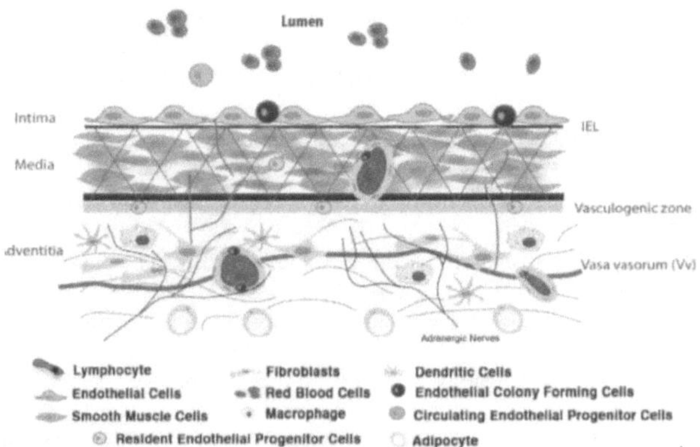

Figure 7: Figure showing cellular composition of the vascular wall with endothelial cells in the intimal layer, smooth muscle cells on the medial layer, and a diverse array of cell types within the adventitial layer. The adventitial layer includes fibroblasts, progenitor cells, immune cells, vasa vasorum, adipocytes, and nerves. This figure aims to provide a comprehensive overview of the cellular diversity present in different layers of the vascular wall, highlighting the intricate composition that contributes to the functional complexity of blood vessels[55]

The adventitial layer is characterized by its abundance in fibroblasts, blood and lymphatic vessels, nerves, progenitor cells, adipocytes and immune cells, rendering it a remarkably heterogeneous compartment within the arterial wall **(Figure 7)** [55]. Cells within the adventitial layer perceive and coordinate responses to a diverse range of stimuli, achieved through intricate communication not only among themselves but also with the cells residing in the medial layer[54,55]. Although various other cell types populate the aorta, it is primarily covered by endothelial cells (ECs), smooth muscle cells (VSMCs), and fibroblasts. The roles of these predominant cell types are detailed below.

2.2.3.1.1 Endothelial Cells

The lumen of blood vessels is lined by a monolayer of endothelial cells, collectively referred to as the endothelium. The endothelium separates the lumen from the tunica media. ECs exhibit polarity with apical and basolateral surfaces, with their apical membrane in contact with the bloodstream, and the basolateral surface in contact with the basement membrane, primarily composed of glycoproteins, non-fibrillar collagens, and other accessory proteins secreted by the ECs themselves[45]. The endothelium plays a crucial role in regulating vascular tone (comprising cyclic contraction and relaxation), as well as controlling the translocation of solutes, fluids, hormones, and macromolecules[56]. Likewise, the endothelium is considered an active metabolic and endocrine organ, particularly because ECs perform essential functions, including a) supplying oxygen to the tissues, b) continuously releasing vasodilatory and vasoconstrictive molecules like NO, and c) initiating signal transduction pathways to regulate reactive species and other metabolites[57]. Disruptions in the delicate balance of such factors can lead to endothelial dysfunction, a condition that underlies various vascular disorders attributed by abnormal vascular remodeling.

2.2.3.1.2 Vascular Smooth Muscle Cells

Different from the ECs, VSMCs play a pivotal role in orchestrating the process of vascular wall ECM remodeling. These spindle-shaped cells, measuring 20-30 μm in length and 4 μm in width, are primarily located within the medial layer of the arterial wall, and in the larger arteries and the aorta are interspersed and in close contact with concentric elastic lamellae. VSMCs can originate from either the mesoderm or the neuroectoderm. However, VSMCs within the vascular tree primarily stem from mesodermal sources, emerging from the mesenchyme during embryonic development or originating from the mesothelium through the process of epithelial-to-mesenchymal transition[58]. The medial VSMCs play an important role maintaining structural integrity of the aorta wall through the production of elastin, collagen, an array of other ECM proteins, as well as various proteases and their inhibitors, VSMCs provide structural integrity to the vessel while also regulating the vessel diameter through contraction and relaxation in response to specific stimuli[49]. Depending on their microenvironment, they can dynamically alter their phenotypes, which enables them to either bolster the extracellular matrix (ECM) components during remodeling or adjust the vascular tone as may be required[49].

VSMCs exhibit a remarkable ability to transition between synthetic proliferative phenotypes and contractile phenotypes (**Figure 8**) depending on their microenvironment. That said, the synthetic and contractile VSMC phenotypes represent theoretical extremes on a phenotypic scale and most VSMCs exhibit characteristics of both. In healthy blood vessels, VSMCs exhibit a more contractile phenotype, characterized by limited ECM protein secretion and abundant myofilament production to allow them to regulate blood vessel diameter and thus blood flow and pressure. This phenotypic plasticity enables VSMCs to perform a regulatory role to maintain vascular tissue homeostasis. VSMCs of a more synthetic phenotype are more prevalent under pathological conditions and are less common or active in healthy tissue milieus. They are associated with cell proliferation, migration, apoptosis, enzyme production, and vascular remodeling[59]. The transition between contractile and synthetic phenotypes is frequently initiated by changes in the spatio-temporal profile of biomolecular factors often initiated by the infiltration of inflammatory and immune cells, and [60,61]. Elevated levels of Il-1β and TNF-α in human AAA biopsies have been observed to influence the shift of VSMCs towards more synthetic phenotypes[62]. Additionally, factors such as reactive oxygen species (ROS) and reactive nitrogen species (RNS) formed due to oxidative metabolism within the cells, because of inflammatory stimuli during injury, and contributions from the adventitial layer, often serve as triggers for this phenotypic transition. Furthermore, the Notch1 pathway is recognized to play a role in AAA formation and VSMC-specific haploinsufficiency of Notch1 promotes contractile VSMC phenotype and prevents matrix remodeling abdominal aorta[63]. Synthetic VSMCs also demonstrate enhanced generation of proteolytic enzymes such as MMPs, the A disintegrin and metalloproteinase (ADAM) family and cathepsins that break down elastic and collagen fibers besides other structural and non-structural protein components of the ECM, and tissue inhibitors of matrix metalloproteases (TIMPs) that serve to counter-act the MMPs to maintain tissue homeostasis[49,64]. Conversely, the contractile VSMCs regulate vascular contraction and relaxation, passively maintaining the appropriate ratio of elastic to collagen to ensure the proper stretch and recoil attributes of the aortal wall[64]. Contractile VSMCs often expresses contractile apparatus proteins such as smooth muscle alpha actin (α-SM-actin or ACTA), smooth muscle myosin heavy chain 2 (SM-MHC-2),and end-stage contractile phenotypic markers such as smoothelin, calponin and vimentin[60].

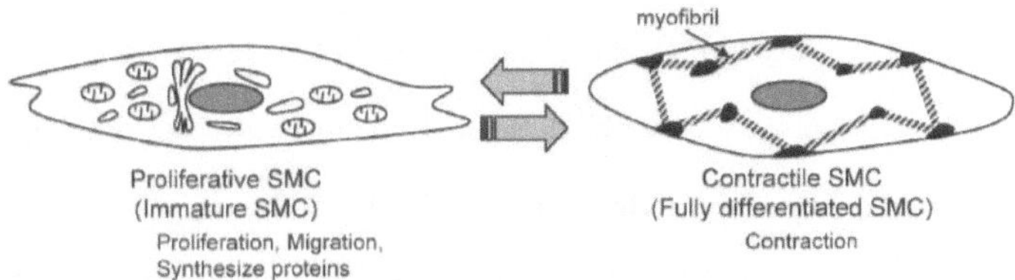

Figure 8: Figure Showing the modulation of contractile and synthetic phenotypes in VSMCs based on the tissue microenvironment. Contractile SMCs represent highly differentiated cell types engaged in continuous contraction and relaxation, crucial for regulating vascular tone. In contrast, synthetic SMCs exhibit heightened proliferation and are involved in synthesizing proteases, including MMPs[60]

Vascular remodeling serves as a mechanism by which tissues eliminate unwanted, aged, or damaged cells, in the process of rearranging structures through cell growth, cell death, cell migration, and degradation or production of ECM proteins[65]. This is a critical adaptive feature required for the maintenance of the blood flow in the vessel wall. Remodeling of the vascular wall is predominantly governed by endothelial cells, VSMCs, fibroblasts, immune cells and is influenced by various factors, including changes in aortal wall tension, shifts in the availability of chemical messengers (such as cytokines specifically TNF-α, IL-1β, IL-4, IL-6, IL-13 etc. and growth factors such as platelet-derived growth factor, epidermal factor, Transforming growth factor beta 1 (TGF-β1) etc.), and alterations in the production of MMPs and or TIMPs[66,67]. While these internal parameters contribute to vascular remodeling, the precise molecular mechanisms that govern this process under such circumstances remain an area of ongoing investigation.

2.2.3.1.3 Fibroblasts

Fibroblasts, the most prevalent cell type in the vascular adventitia, originate from primary mesenchyme, local epithelial-mesenchymal transition (EMT), and bone marrow-derived precursors[55]. Their primary role is to impart mechanical strength to the tissue by secreting essential extracellular matrix (ECM) components, most notably fibrillar collagen, including Type I and III collagen, thus forming a supportive framework within the aorta. A notable characteristic shared with VSMCs is the fibroblasts' ability to differentiate into myofibroblast phenotypes, expressing smooth muscle alpha-actin (α-SM-actin), which is predominantly observed in VSMCs with contractile characteristics[55,68]. These myofibroblasts play a crucial role in tissue remodeling due to their multifaceted physiological functions in response to changes in the local environment. They contribute to the production of various ECM components, such as collagen, elastin, fibronectin, as well as matricellular proteins like tenascin-C and osteopontin[69]. Additionally, they release a variety of growth factors, cytokines, and reactive oxygen species (ROS) that exert paracrine effects on the VSMCs located in the medial layer[55]. Furthermore, fibroblasts possess the capability to migrate from the adventitial layer to the medial or intimal layer, thereby contributing to the pathological remodeling of the aortic wall.

2.2.3.2 ECM Components

The lamellar unit, serving as the fundamental structural building block within the aortic media, encompasses two elastic lamellae that envelop VSMCs and the extracellular matrix (ECM). This intricate arrangement plays a crucial role in maintaining the integrity and functionality of the vasculature. The medial layer of the aorta comprises parallel arrangements of these lamellar units, providing the entropic elasticity necessary for the vessel to stretch and recoil in response to the pulsatile forces generated by blood flow[70,71].

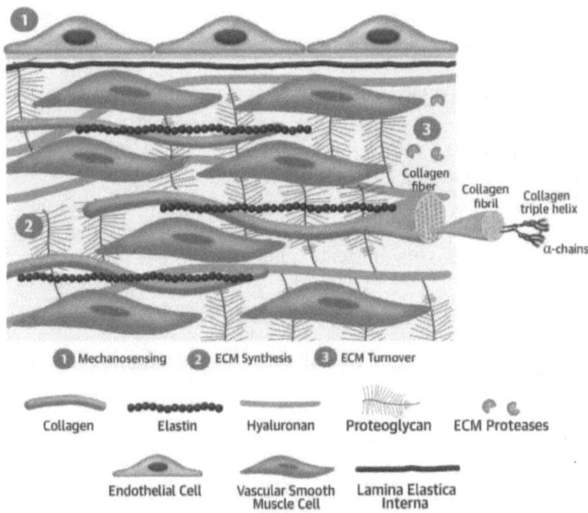

Figure 9: Key elements of the aortal ECM including elastic fibers, collagens, and proteoglycans. Emphasizing their significance, the figure illustrates their roles in physiological regulation. Endothelial cells and SMCs are depicted as key players in mechanosensing, responding to alterations in ECM components. This mechanosensing is crucial for ECM synthesis, turnover, and overall homeostasis[71]

Mature vessel wall ECM is a complex arrangement of fibrous proteins, associated with glycoproteins embedded in a hydrated ground substance of glycosaminoglycans and proteoglycans. The ECM, a specialized three-dimensional network of macromolecules produced by cells within the medial layer, plays a vital role in aortic physiology. In the ECM, there is a thin layer of highly specialized basement membrane that connects cells from the matrix microenvironment and is a reservoir for growth factors, chemical messengers, and cytokines that regulate their bioavailability and cell functions[72]. It consists primarily of glycoproteins, proteoglycans and glycosaminoglycans (e.g. hyaluronan), and fibrillar proteins collagen and elastin (**Figure 9**) [73]. These molecular components are instrumental in mediating essential cell signaling processes, determining cell fate, and orchestrating vessel wall remodeling. The precise organization and composition of the lamellar unit and ECM within the aortic media are paramount for maintaining proper vascular function. This intricate interplay ensures the aorta's ability to withstand the dynamic forces of blood flow, regulate vascular tone, and engage in critical signaling processes that contribute to overall vessel health and homeostasis.

2.2.3.2.1 Glycoproteins

Glycoproteins, comprised of both protein and carbohydrate components, exert a crucial influence on the structure, function, and health of arteries. Found within the ECM and cell membranes, glycoproteins serve to maintain vascular integrity and to modulate cellular interactions in the vessel wall. They facilitate cell-matrix adhesion and signaling, playing a pivotal role in cell migration, proliferation, and tissue remodeling[74]. Glycoproteins participate and facilitate assembly and organization of the ECM, ensuring proper tissue architecture and function. Cell membrane-associated glycoproteins are integral to various cellular processes within the arterial wall. They participate in cell adhesion, enabling cells to adhere to the vessel wall and to each other, which is critical for maintaining tissue cohesion and vascular integrity[74]. Additionally, glycoproteins are involved in signal transduction pathways, mediating communication between cells and their microenvironment. Laminin and fibronectin are the best studied glycoproteins of the ECM of the vascular wall. Laminin, a heterotrimer composed of three polypeptide subunits, holds a unique position. It forges bonds with other ECM proteins and, in a self-organized manner, forms an intricately cross-linked web-like structure intertwined with collagen type IV fibers, crafting a specialized basement membrane[74]. This proximity facilitates cell attachment via cell surface receptors (integrins and non-integrins), making laminin indispensable for embryonic development and embryogenesis[75].

Differently, fibronectin is a versatile glycoprotein that functions as an interlink between cells and the ECM. Secreted as a large dimeric glycoprotein with subunits ranging in size from 230 kDa to 270 kDa, fibronectin harbors binding domains for numerous ECM proteins and carbohydrates[76,77]. Within arteries, fibronectin establishes vital connections with cells by binding to cell surface receptors and ECM constituents, including collagen and integrins, thereby governing cellular adhesion. This intricate interaction proves pivotal for cell anchoring and migration, especially during critical processes like tissue repair and vessel remodeling. Similar to laminin, fibronectin also undergoes self-assembly, facilitated by the amino-terminal domain that plays a pivotal role in collagen fibrillogenesis[78]. Additionally, fibronectin engages in regulating cell signaling pathways, influencing cell behavior, encompassing proliferation and differentiation, thereby contributing to maintenance of arterial homeostasis and repair[77].

Together, laminin and fibronectin support cell attachment, migration, and signaling, all of which are essential for arterial development, maintenance, and response to various physiological and pathological stimuli. Thus, abnormalities in expression or structure of laminin and fibronectin can contribute to pathophysiology of vascular disorders such as atherosclerosis and arterial fibrosis.

2.2.3.2.2 Proteoglycans and Glycosaminoglycans

Proteoglycans (PGs) are key ECM components comprised of a core protein covalently attached to multiple glycosaminoglycans (GAGs), long-chain polysaccharides[79]. The polysaccharide chains of the PGs are hydrophilic and help in binding to water thereby hydrating the entire ECM and providing turgor to the matrix. This provides a shock absorbing and compression resisting ability to the ECM and therefore are widely responsible for pressure dissipation particularly in arterial wall and cartilages[79]. Most PGs are present in the medial layer of the arterial wall and are often associated with elastin, collagen and cells. However, PGs can be found at different locations in the arterial wall, but their functions are largely determined by the GAGs that are attached to it[80].

GAGs are the most negatively charged linear and unbranched macromolecules with repeating disaccharide units[81]. These biologically active sugars, also termed glycans, intertwine with proteins to create proteoglycans, thereby introducing functional diversity to proteins[81,82]. GAGs exhibit independent functions, significantly influencing the structural and functional facets of arterial tissues. They engage in both reversible and irreversible interactions with positively charged matrix components, including proteins and

growth factors[83]. Their interaction with collagen and elastin, for instance, is pivotal in

Table 1: Summary of PGs and their associated GAGs[84]

PG	GAGs	Location in the aorta	Role
Versican	Chondroitin sulfate (CS)	Throughout the aorta in the medial layer concentrated in regions rich in VSMCs	Provides support for proliferation and migration of VSMCs
Biglycan	Chondroitin sulfate (CS)/Dermatan sulfate (DS)	Present within intimal thickening, plaques, and fibrous cap	facilitates lipoprotein retention
Decorin	Chondroitin sulfate (CS)/Dermatan sulfate (DS)	Adventitial layer of both normal and atherosclerotic arteries, and within the intima of arteries that resist atherosclerosis	Stabilizes plaque stability
Perlecan	Heparin/Heparan sulfate	Mostly abundant in mice at the basement membrane between endothelial cells and VSMCs	Acts as a permeability barrier in mice, no clear function in humans

modulating overall mechanical properties of the arterial wall. This intricate and highly

specialized protein-sugar interplay regulates wide ranges of protein functions influenced

by the precise composition of proteins and sugars within the ECM. Furthermore, GAGs act

as binding sites for growth factors and cytokines, thus steering their availability and

interactions with cells. Despite comprising a mere 1-5% of the total ECM composition,

GAGs wield substantial influence over protein functionality, enhancing their roles within

arterial tissues[85]. In addition, In the arterial ECM, GAGs contribute substantially to both

hydration and mechanical attributes of the vascular wall. Their innate hydrophilicity enables them to attract water molecules, culminating in a hydrated gel-like matrix that endows the arterial wall with compression resistance and the capability to withstand mechanical forces arising from blood flow[86]. This facet is pivotal for preserving the arterial wall's resilience and structural integrity.

The distinct assembly of sugars within the GAGs introduces plasticity to GAGs. Based on their core, disaccharide structure, GAGs are subdivided into chondroitin sulfate (CS)/dermatan sulfate (DS), heparin/heparan sulfate (HS), keratan sulfate, and hyaluronan, also known as hyaluronic acid. Except hyaluronan, secreted within the plasma membrane, all GAGs are produced in endoplasmic reticulum (ER) and Golgi apparatus[87]. **Table 1** provides an overview of the different proteoglycans and their associated GAG chains[84].

2.2.3.2.3 Collagen

Collagen stands as a vital load-bearing element within the vascular wall's extracellular matrix (ECM). It adopts a fibrillar form and emerges from the intricate arrangement of three polypeptide strands, referred to as α-strands. These chains feature a left-handed helix conformation that intertwines to form a remarkable triple helix structure. The stability of this triple helix is fortified by numerous hydrogen bonds, fostering the creation of covalent bonds that crosslink within the helices. This resultant aggregated structure is known as tropocollagen, serving as the building block of collagen fiber. Elastic fibers and fibrillar collagen comprise an approx. of 50% of the dry weight of larger arteries and almost 80-90% of the collagen present in the arteries are principally fibrillar collagen type I and Type III. These collagen types constitute the major constituents of the intima, media, and adventitia layers. The remaining collagen types form only a fraction of the overall collagen composition[73]. Collagen type III imparts extensile properties to the arterial wall, working in harmony with the network of other collagen types to bestow structural integrity and tensile characteristics[52,88]. Collagen Type IV and type V are found within the endothelial and the basement membranes alongside collagen type I and type III[89]. Collagen's role within the aortic wall's ECM is paramount, its architectural configuration and content undergoing alterations due to aging, hormonal influences, and pathological conditions. For instance, aging is associated with a stiffer aortic wall, potentially linked to changes in wall stresses imposed by blood flow and alterations in the chemical composition of the aortic structure. Notably, collagen concentration rises relative to other fibrillar proteins within the aortic ECM, exacerbating stiffening and elevating the risk of rupture[90].

2.2.3.2.4 Elastin and Elastic Fibers

Elastic fibers, comprised of elastin, a hydrophobic fibrillar structural ECM protein as a key component, confers stretch and recoil properties to the vessel. During cardiac systole, when the heart pumps out blood, the elastic matrix in the aorta wall allows the vessel to expand to accommodate the blood. The kinetic energy of the blood is transferred to the vessel wall and stored as elastic energy. During cardiac diastole, when the heart is filling with blood, blood pressure in the arterial tree is maintained by elastic recoil of the aorta wall transferring this potential energy to blood as kinetic energy to propel it forward, thus maintaining blood pressure. This is known as the *Windkessel effect*[91].

In humans, elastin represents 20-50% of the total dry weight of the aorta tissue[92]. The elastic component is secreted by the specialized VSMCs and fibroblasts in the form of soluble elastin, tropoelastin (approx. 70 kDa), which undergoes complex assembly journey and crosslinking activated by an enzyme called lysyl oxidase (LOX) ultimately culminating in the formation of resilient elastic fibers, comprised of a core of amorphous, crosslinked elastin deposited on a pre-scaffold of glycoprotein-based microfibrils (**Figure 10**)[93]. However, in pathological conditions such as AAAs, there is a notable breakdown and loss of elastic matrix in the aorta wall and thus reduced content relative to collagen. This alteration renders the arterial wall less elastic and stiffer compared to the normal value of modulus of elasticity ($0.7\text{-}40 \times 10^6$ dynes/cm^2)[94]. Such changes not only compromise the vessel's capacity to efficiently stretch and recoil but also adversely impact vascular VSMC phenotype and behavior since elastic fibers closely modulate these responses by modulating cell-matrix interaction ultimately activating transduction pathways within VSMCs[95,96].

2.2.3.2.5 Assembly of elastic fibers and collagen fibers

Elastic fibers and collagen fibers are the major structural ECM components of the aorta wall. They undergo continuous remodeling over a lifetime, to critically maintain the structural and functional integrity of the aorta wall. Elastin, a highly stable and hydrophobic biopolymer, imparts elasticity and resilience to arteries. These elastic fibers comprises predominantly 90% (of the fiber) of elastin protein, and 10% of elastin associated glycoproteins, including fibrillins, fibulins and emilins[97]. Due to its high level of crosslinking and hydrophobicity owing to a high content of hydrophobic amino acids, which contributes to its high resistance to degradation in aqueous environments, elastin has a long half-life of 60-70 years[98]. Also, due to the crosslinking between adjacent elastin molecules, elastic fibers possess a remarkable capacity to stretch up to eight times their original length and yet elastically retract when the stretching forces are removed.

The process of de novo elastic fiber assembly, termed as elastogenesis, is a complex, multi-step process involving elastin precursor (tropoelastin) synthesis, coacervation, cross-linking, engagement with glycoprotein pre-scaffolds, and further amalgamation and extension of elastin deposits to form fibers. In the aortal wall, VSMCs and to a lesser extent, fibroblasts, synthesize elastin precursors which are later transported outside onto the cell surface (**Figure 10**). There is some evidence that ECs are also capable of elastin synthesis, although this is rather limited even in healthy tissues[48,99,100]. Tropoelastin is primarily synthesized during perinatal development although its synthesis can be prompted later in response to tissue remodeling[101]. Tropoelastin undergoes self-assembly when it engages with the elastin binding protein (EBP) on the cell surface. The coacervation of tropoelastin is an endothermic and entropically favorable process and self-assembly, which is temperature dependant results in an n-mer structure. The tropoelastin molecule contains alternating hydrophobic (b-sheet) and hydrophilic (a-helical) domains and the hydrophobic domain is responsible for coacervation. Briefly, the elastin molecule is comprised of repeat sequences of non-polar amino acids such as valine, glycine, alanine, and (VGVAPG), which account for 82% of the entire AA sequence. Mostly located in the β-sheet domains they contribute to protein folding influenced by their unfavorable interactions with water[101,102]. At higher temperatures, these hydrophobic domains permit the self-aggregation of tropoelastin molecules. After the coacervation of the tropoelastin, the lysine residue of the hydrophilic domain participates in crosslinking between adjacent tropoelastin molecules. Lysyl oxidase (LOX) and lysine oxidase like (LOXL) enzymes convert amino group of the lysine residues to aminoadipic and allysine[103]. These intermediates crosslinks through aldol condensation to form bifunctional crosslinks that can undergo further condensation to form desmosine and isodesmosine linkages[47]. Once these complex structures have been formed, they are deposited onto the microfibril scaffold of elastic fibers comprised of the glycoproteins fibrillin 1, fibulin 4 and fibulin 5. Fibrillin stabilizes tropoelastin whereas fibulins bind LOX and fibrillin-1 to spatially coordinate the formation of crosslinked, alkali-insoluble elastic fibers[104].

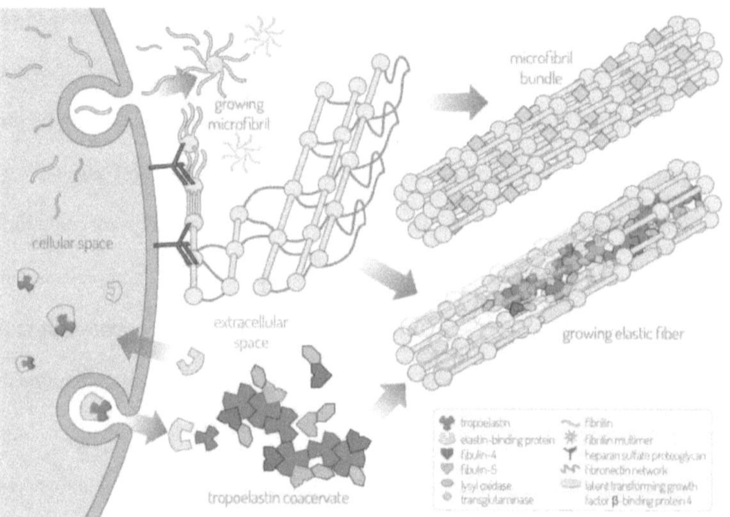

Figure 10. Schematic illustration of microfibril and elastic fiber formation[100]. The upper part of the figure shows multimerization of fibrillin molecules and subsequent formation of crosslinked microfibril with participation of various proteins and association processes. The lower part demonstrates the simple process of formation and coacervation of tropoelastin into fibrillin microfibril eventually leading to forming elastic fibers through crosslinking with the help of various matrix molecules

Unlike elastin, the lifespan of vascular collagen is much shorter, at ~60-70 days[105]. Collagens exhibit a trimeric composition with repeating sequences of Glycine-proline-hydroxyproline. This distinctive triad arrangement of collagens gives rise to a helical conformation that intertwines with two additional helices, creating a triple-helical structure. Initially, vascular cells synthesize collagen in the form of pre-procollagen, which is then translocated to the endoplasmic reticulum (ER)[106]. Within the ER, chaperones, and enzymes like prolyl and lysyl hydroxylase contribute to folding and trimerization, yielding a thermodynamically stable procollagen with non-helical end groups rich in disulfide bonds. In the extracellular matrix (ECM), these disulfide bonds undergo cleavage, resulting in the formation of an insoluble tropocollagen structure[106]. Tropocollagen molecules align themselves to construct collagen fibrils, subsequently undergoing crosslinking by lysyl oxidase to culminate in the formation of fully mature and crosslinked collagen fibers[107].

2.2.4   ECM Remodeling

Vascular remodeling is a pivotal adaptive process integral to fetal development and growth[65] on one hand, and the tissue adaptation in adult vessels post-injury. This natural phenomenon encompasses essential structural modifications with implications to cell proliferation, migration, apoptosis, as well as the synthesis and degradation of the extracellular matrix in response to chemical and biomechanical changes to the vascular microenvironment[95]. Vascular remodeling is enabled by endothelial and smooth muscle cells, and fibroblasts as an adaptation response to signal transduction incited by altered mechanical and hemodynamic stimuli, and growth factors[95,108]. However, remodeling can frequently take on an undesirable trajectory to culminate in pathological alterations to the vessel wall, as seen in atherosclerotic plaque development and arteriosclerosis. While atherosclerosis is marked by a localized inflammatory reaction within the intima due to lipid accumulation in plaques, arteriosclerosis represents a broader, diffuse modification of the medial layer of arterial blood vessels. Arteriosclerosis is typically linked to the aging process and widespread cardiovascular, metabolic, or inflammatory disorders. Over time, it can lead to irreversible deterioration of the extracellular matrix, potentially compromising the overall health of the vascular system.

2.2.4.1 Extracellular Proteolytic System and its Regulation

The composition and integrity of the extracellular matrix (ECM) plays an important role in shaping the physical and functional attributes of the aorta wall. The vascular ECM undergoes continuous remodeling to replace aged and non-functional components with fully intact and functional proteins. This process is orchestrated by the proteolytic/protease system present within the ECM of the aorta wall. Among these enzymes, MMPs are particularly abundant and active, though other serine and cysteine proteases, such as cathepsins, contribute to degradation and turnover of specific ECM proteins.

MMPs constitute a family of zinc-containing calcium-dependent endopeptidases, also known as matrixins. They are synthesized by various cell types including VSMCs, macrophages, neutrophils, lymphocytes, ECs, and fibroblasts[95,109]. These MMPs are often produced as transmembrane proteins, anchored by proteoglycans such as heparan sulfate glycosaminoglycans[110]. MMPs are mostly secreted in an inactive (zymogen) form and are activated later through proteolytic cleavage of the N-terminal pro-domain. Categorized based on substrate specificity as collagenases, gelatinases, stromelysins, and matrilysins, the enzyme activities of the MMPs are controlled at the transcriptional level, and zymogen activation, specific protein interactions (as detailed in the **Table 2**), and enzyme inhibition are controlled by intrinsic inhibitors like the tissue inhibitors of MMPs (TIMPs) **(Table 3)**[111]. MMPs significantly contribute to tissue remodeling, wound healing, angiogenesis, and tumor invasion due to their proteolytic activity[112]. They also modulate cellular processes such as migration, proliferation, and survival, alongside influencing the activation of other MMPs and cytokines like TNF-α etc[110,113].

Table 2: List of MMPs[111]

Subclass	MMP Type	Substrate
Collagenases	MMP1, MMP8, MMP13, MMP18	Collagen Types I, II, III
Gelatinases	MMP2, MMP9	Collagen I, III, IV, V, Elastin, basement membrane, gelatin
Stromelysins	MMP3, MMP10, MMP11, MMP19, MMP20	Laminin, fibronectin, non-helical collagen, Collagen IV, gelatin
Membrane-Type (MT-MMPs)	MMP14, MMP15, MMP16, MMP17	Collagen Type I, II, III, gelatin,
Human Macrophage Metalloprotease	MMP12	Elastin, fibronectin
Other: Matrilysin	MMP7	Laminin, fibronectin, collagens (non-fibrillar)

Cathepsins are a group of cysteine proteases, that contribute to the degradation and turnover of the structural proteins cleaving mostly elastin, collagen, and other ECM components, thereby influencing the mechanical properties of the aorta wall[114]. Excessive production and/or dysregulation of these proteases is detrimental to vascular integrity and contributes to the pathophysiology of vascular disorders such as aneurysms.

The activation and proteolytic activity of MMPs are regulated by TIMPS. Maintaining a balanced MMP/TIMP ratio is pivotal to coordinating matrix production, maturation, and degradation. TIMPs form non-covalent 1:1 stoichiometric complexes with MMPs, effectively inactivating them[115]. Four TIMPs (TIMP1, TIMP2, TIMP3, TIMP4) have been identified in vertebrates, which can sometimes tissue specific but often inhibits all MMPs[116]. Within the aortic wall VSMCs and ECs produce MMPs and TIMPs, notably MMP2 and MMP9 take center stage in proteolytic remodeling, while all TIMPs work to counter MMPs, preserving the equilibrium between matrix degradation and production.

Table 3: Role of TIMPs[116]

Family member	Reported Function
TIMP1	Inhibits of all MMPs. Associates with proMMP9. Inhibits angiogenesis.
TIMP2	Inhibits of all MMPs. Associates with MT1-MMP and MMP2 at cell surface and regulates MMP2 activation.
TIMP3	Inhibits of all MMPs. Extracellular matrix-associated
TIMP4	Inhibits of all MMPs

2.2.4.2 Role of Signal Transduction Pathways

In the vascular wall, bioactive molecules bind to diverse cell surface receptors, initiating intracellular signal transduction cascades. These internal signals orchestrate fundamental cellular processes, spanning gene transcription, protein synthesis, cytoskeletal rearrangement, endocytosis, cellular metabolism, proliferation, migration, apoptosis, and survival. Upon engagement with these extracellular cues, signal transduction is activated within the cell. MAPK signaling and NO signaling are two paramount and ubiquitous pathways that regulate a spectrum of cellular and extracellular matrix properties within the artery wall.

MAPKs comprise a cluster of serine/threonine protein kinases that regulate a variety of diverse intracellular and extracellular responses. Noteworthy among them are the ERK and JNK, which fall within the stress-activated protein kinases (SAPK) category[117]. These kinases play pivotal roles in a range of biological processes, encompassing cell proliferation, differentiation, metabolism, motility, and the survival and apoptosis of VSMCs, thereby exerting significant influence on various facets of vascular remodeling. The disruption of these cascades is central to the etiology of several tissue disorders.

An equally critical regulator of vascular ECM homeostasis is NO, a naturally occurring molecule that serves a vital role in modulating platelet aggregation, leukocyte-endothelium adhesion, vascular tone, and phenotypic modulation of vascular VSMCs[46]. NO is synthesized from L-arginine in endothelial cells through calcium-calmodulin dependent enzymatic activity[46]. Maintaining adequate NO levels is integral to preserving normal vascular physiology. Diminished NO bioavailability and endothelial dysfunction, however, are linked to the development of diseases such as atherosclerosis, hypertension, hypercholesterolemia, diabetes, congestive heart failure, and thrombosis, all of which are directly or indirectly associated with aneurysms[46]. Both the MAPK and NO signaling pathways orchestrate the transcriptional regulation of vascular remodeling processes. Notably, they govern the production of MMPs, cytokines, and inflammatory and anti-inflammatory responses. The comprehensive roles of MAPKs and NO are further explored in sections 2.4 and 2.5.

2.2.4.3 Abnormalities of the elastic matrix

Despite its prolonged half-life and slow turnover rate, the elastic matrix undergoesgradual degradation, thereby compromising the structural integrity of the vascular wall. This deterioration results from a combination of intrinsic and extrinsic factors. Intrinsic aging of the vascular wall is attributed to factors such as natural aging, hereditary influences, elevated blood pressure, lipid accumulation, calcification, and enzymatic responses. At the molecular level, intrinsic aging may be initiated by a range of factors, including proteolytic (enzymatic) degradation, oxidative damage, aspartic acid racemization, lipid binding and accumulation, carbamylation, the formation of advanced glycation end products (AGEs), and mechanical fatigue resulting from wall stress, among others. In contrast, extrinsic factors encompass smoking, UV exposure, and imbalanced diets. The interplay of these diverse factors significantly contributes to aberrations in elastic fibers, culminating in mechanical fatigue and severe pathologies.

This intricate scenario is further complicated by the enzymatic breakdown of elastin, facilitated by the constitutive expression of proteases. These enzymes, when unleashed due to the combined impact of the aforementioned factors, can lead to impairment or even loss of elastic fiber functionality. This degradation process also results in the release of degraded elastin peptides, also known as elastokines[100], which possess bioactive properties and actively participate in inflammatory responses. The proteolytic damage to elastic fibers, accompanied by the influence of elastokines, plays a critical role in the emergence of grave pathological conditions. These conditions encompass a wide range, from lung emphysema and atherosclerosis to chronic obstructive pulmonary disease (COPD), aneurysms, and even UV-induced photoaging[100].

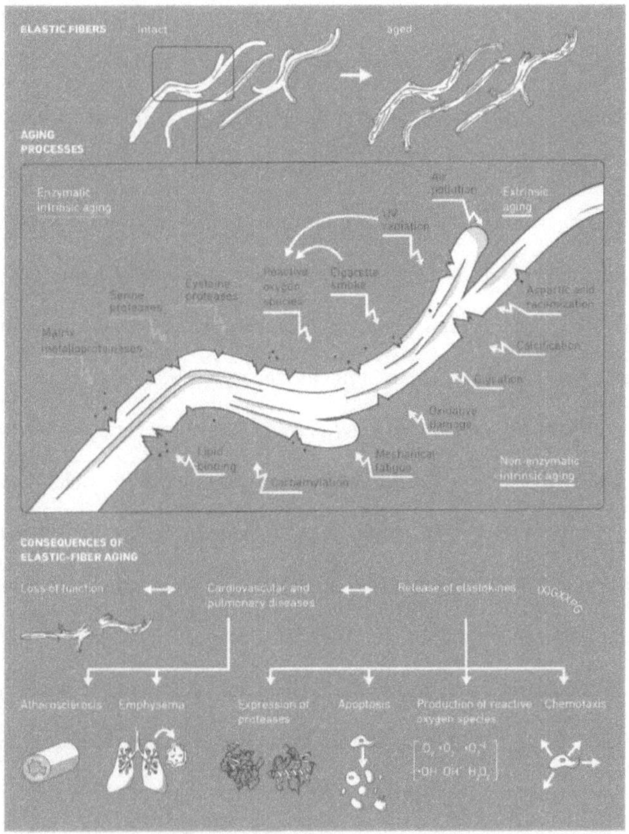

Figure 11: Factors associated with vascular aging and elastic fiber deterioration. Elastic fibers are exposed to various factors over a span of time that results in many pathological conditions leading to the loss of function of the elastic fibers[100]

2.3 Abdominal Aortic Aneurysms

2.3.1 Definition, Risk Factors and Aortic Dissection

An aortal or arterial aneurysm represents an irreversible localized expansion of the vessel wall, stretching to a diameter at least 1.5 times larger than the typical vessel diamater[118]. Aneurysms are multifocal and can manifest at various locations throughout the body. The abdominal aorta traverses the diaphragm and continues downward between the kidneys. Notably, arterial aneurysms tend to materialize most frequently within the abdominal aorta, especially in the segment positioned beneath the kidneys immediately after the aorta divides to create the renal arteries (renal bifurcation). These particular aneurysms are identified as infrarenal aneurysms[119].

The emergence of an AAA can stem from several factors that contribute to the disruption and loss of structural proteins within the aortic wall. These structural proteins, primarily collagen and elastic fibers provide vital support and stability to the vessel's structure. While the precise cause remains not entirely elucidated, atherosclerosis, characterized by the accumulation of plaque comprising fatty substances, cholesterol, cellular debris, calcium, and fibrin along the inner lining of an artery, is believed to be a major risk factor for AAA development. The other risk factors for development of AAAs are age (greater than 50 years), male (occurs more frequently in male than females), genetic predisposition, hyperlipidemia, hypertension, smoking and diabetes[120]. While the risk of AAA formation is lower in women than in men, AAA rupture in females aortas occur more rapidly than in males[7].

The feared and often fatal complication of AAA is rupture, where the aneurysm wall experiences structural failure, resulting in extensive retro- and/or intraperitoneal hemorrhage. Rupture risk is closely linked to the size of the aneurysm, with the aneurysm diameter serving as a pivotal indicator. The likelihood of rupture significantly rises when the aortic diameter exceeds 5.5 cm (5 cm in females). The cumulative rupture rate for incidentally diagnosed aneurysms in population-based studies within five years ranges from 25% to 40% for aneurysms larger than 5.0 cm, while rupture carries a mortality rate exceeding 80%[121,122]. Left untreated, aortic rupture is invariably fatal, with over half of affected patients succumbing prior to reaching medical care.

2.3.2 Diagnosis and Screening

AAAs pose a diagnostic challenge due to their asymptomatic nature, making their initial detection and screening complex. Often, they are incidentally identified during clinical abdominal examinations for unrelated reasons, employing methods like computed tomography (CT), magnetic resonance imaging (MRI), or ultrasound. One fundamental diagnostic approach involves assessing the aortic diameter, measured from either outer-to-outer or inner-to-inner (both <30 mm for normal aorta), particularly monitoring if it surpasses 30 mm through ultrasonography. Contrast-enhanced CT scans can help differentiate healthy arteries from those with coexisting aneurysms by revealing anatomical variations in the aorta and arteries. Despite efforts, effectively preventing the progression of AAAs remains elusive, likely due to their intricate pathogenesis involving a diverse array of peptides, proteins, enzymes, and cells. The U.S. Preventive Services Task Force (USPSTF) recommends a one-time screening for AAAs in men aged 65 and above, especially those with a history of smoking, to mitigate premature mortality risks. Additionally, women who are current smokers and possess a higher familial prevalence of AAAs are also advised to undergo a one-time screening to identify any concurrent aneurysms[123].

2.3.3   Current standard of Care

2.3.3.1   Managing AAA Progression: Current Strategies and the Need for Innovative New Approaches

The primary step in managing AAA involves quitting smoking, a major risk factor for AAAs. This action has the potential to decelerate the progression of AAAs and mitigate the risk of fatal rupture, even among patients with existing AAAs. Given the substantial fatality rate of over 80% associated with AAAs, adopting a healthful diet and regular monitoring of aortic diameter changes becomes crucial. Nevertheless, despite vigilant dietary choices, reversing AAA pathophysiology once initiated is generally unattainable.

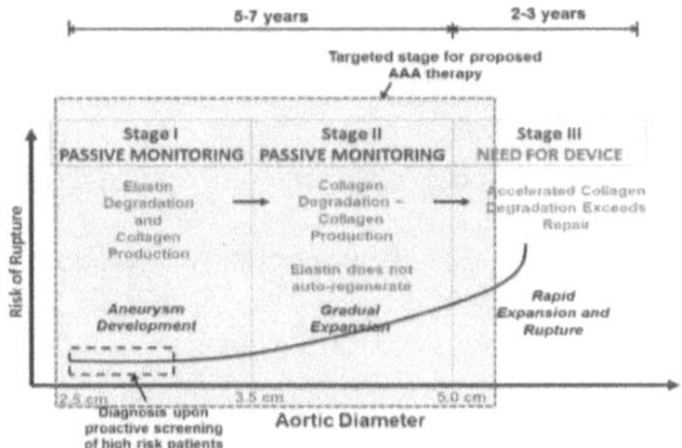

Figure 12: Schematic showing current management of AAAs, delineated into three stages of progression. Stages I and II, the initiation phase, involves passive monitoring of detected aneurysms for growth, marked by substantial degradation of both elastin and collagen. While collagen can be actively reproduced by vascular smooth muscle cells (vSMCs), elastin degradation is less readily addressed. Stage III signifies severe AAAs, characterized by accelerated deterioration of both elastin and collagen, necessitating surgical intervention for effective management

At present, there exists no effective treatment for small AAAs (diameter 30<d<5.5 cm) except for routine screening of high-risk patients through methods such as ultrasound,

MRI, or CT. The development of small AAAs unfolds in two stages. This process encompasses the initial degradation of elastic fibers and collagen fibers, followed by a phase of compensatory collagen regeneration that seeks to offset the loss of elastic fibers, which is naturally irreversible **(Figure 12)**.

With no proven drug-based treatments, AAAs that have exceeded a critical size for rupture (> 5.5 cm) are mostly surgically treated through either open surgical repair or endovascular aneurysm repair (EVAR)[124]. On a molecular level, at this stage, both elastin and collagen degradation are chronic and significant. Compensatory mechanisms are constrained resulting in a low elastic matrix to collagen ratio. Consequently, AAAs at this stage become highly susceptible to rupture, which is why one of the two elective surgical approaches is typically recommended. Open surgical repair encompasses procedures such as transperitoneal or left peritoneal incisions, followed by the insertion of a tube-shaped graft into the aorta. This graft is then enveloped around the aneurysmal sac of the aorta and sutured **(Figure 13A)**, but this invasive technique might not be suitable for elderly individuals due to its complexity and associated higher perioperative risks[125]. The serious risks include hemorrhage, multiple organ dysfunction syndrome related to reperfusion following aortic clamping[126].

In contrast, EVAR has emerged as a minimally invasive alternative, demonstrating better post-operative outcomes in terms of mortality and morbidity. This approach involves accessing the circulation through femoral arteries and inserting a stent into a catheter, which is then guided to the aneurysmal site. Upon placement of the stent at the site, normal blood flow is restored **(Figure 13B)**[127]. However, potential complications such as endoleaks, stent migration, and intimal hyperplasia are associated with EVAR, can lead to stent graft failure[127]. Consequently, there is a crucial demand for innovative non-surgical treatment strategies that can halt or even reverse the growth of AAAs over the extended timeline of their growth to a high-risk rupture stage. Such treatments would be highly significant in reducing the need for surgical intervention in the mostly high-risk elderly patient demographic.

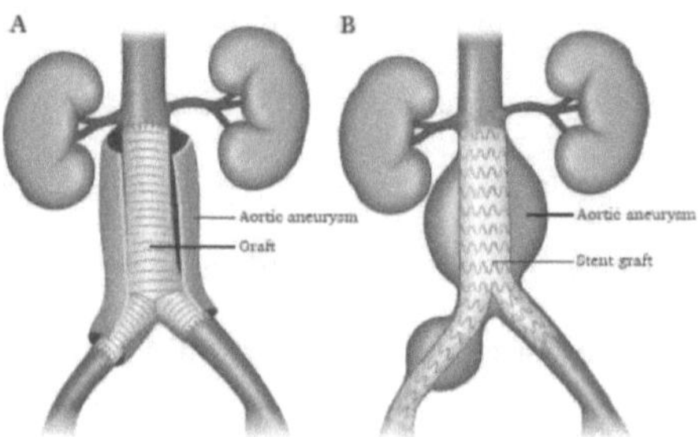

Figure 13: Surgical strategies for treating AAAs involve graft deployment in the affected region[128]. (A) Open surgical repair entails a highly invasive intervention. (B) Endovascular aneurysm repair (EVAR) represents a minimally invasive technique

2.3.3.2   Drug-Based Strategies to treat Small AAAs

Various drug-based treatment strategies have been explored to potentially slow down the progression of small AAA (<5.5 cm), with limited success. Medications like statins, although lacking definitive evidence of their effectiveness in preventing AAA growth, are widely used for their anti-inflammatory, anti-oxidative, and anti-proteolytic properties. Experimental investigations demonstrate that atorvastatin, cerivastatin, and simvastatin can diminish proteolytic degradation of the elastic matrix by reducing MMPs, particularly MMP9, in *in-vivo* and *ex-vivo* models, suggesting potential benefits in curtailing elastic matrix damage[129]. As mounting evidence associates angiotensin II with AAA formation, angiotensin-converting enzyme (ACE) inhibitors (captopril, lisinopril, enalapril) and angiotensin II receptor blockers (ARBs) (losartan) are have been delivered to manage the inflammation-related cellular effect on macrophage infiltration and ROS due to hypertension on the AAA wall[129]. Some studies have suggested that losartan enhances TGF-β signaling to suppress MMP-dependent elastic matrix degradation[130]. Antibiotics like doxycycline (DOX) and Rapamycin have demonstrated potential in reducing AAA expansion alongside decreased MMP9 expression[131]. Apart from the drugs listed above, other alternative pharmacological drugs have also been tested based on their target which are listed in the **Table 4**. Despite the range of drugs employed in AAA management, many have failed to present promising outcomes in halting or reversing AAA pathophysiology. This is partially attributed to limited randomized clinical trials and small sample sizes.

Table 4: Table summarizing other pharmacotherapies and their mechanism of inhibiting AAAs

Drug	Target	Model used	Mechanism of AAA inhibition	Reference
A-Tocopherol (Vitamin E)	Oxidative stress	Elastase/Rat	ROS ↓ ,macrophage infiltration ↓	132
17β-estradiol	Estrogen receptor	Elastase/Rat	Macrophage infiltration ↓ , MCP-1 ↓ , NF-κB activity ↓ , MMP9 ↓ , preserved elastin	133
Pyrrolidine dithiocarbamate (PDTC)	NF-κβ	Elastase/mice	Mast cell and macrophage infiltration ↓ , IFN-γ ↓ , IL-6 ↓ , MMP activity ↓ , preserved elastin	134

2.3.4 Pathophysiology of AAAs

AAAs are complex conditions resulting from the interplay of multiple pathophysiological processes that collectively lead to the naturally irreversible degradation and loss of the aortal wall elastic matrix and gradual wall weakening to fatal rupture (**Figure 14**). The structural integrity of the aorta is intimately tied to its constituent structural ECM components, and any alterations to these components can compromise its integrity. Key among these components are the fibrous proteins, primarily elastin and collagen, which provide both compliance and tensile strength to the abdominal aorta. However, as age and inflammation increase, the degradation of these fibrous proteins occurs, initiating and advancing AAAs.

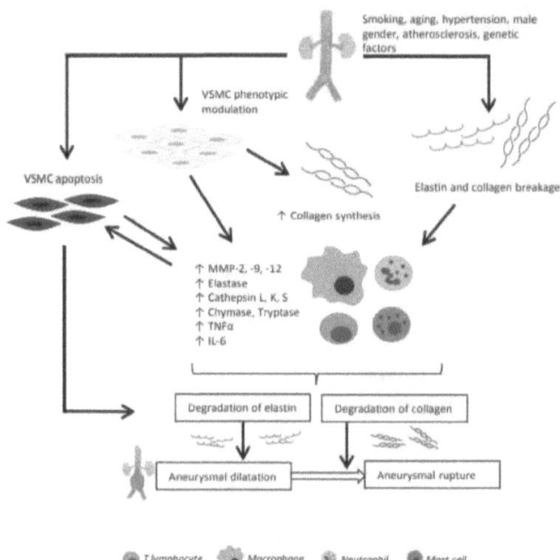

Figure 14: Simplified overview of pathogenesis of AAAs illustrating the sequence of events. The diagram highlights vSMCs ability to produce MMPs when stimulated by risk factors and induce degradation of elastin and collagen, ultimately contributing to AAA formation[135]

Despite extensive research focused on understanding AAAs in humans, the precise triggers for aneurysm formation remain elusive. Determining the exact influence of any etiological factor has proven challenging, primarily due to the absence of a reliable AAA model. The molecular and cellular mechanisms underlying this disease are still not fully elucidated. Nevertheless, it is evident that the pathogenesis involves several key factors: (a) the infiltration of immune cells into the aneurysmal site, (b) the activation of macrophages and surrounding VSMCs to produce MMPs, (c) the degradation of both elastin and collagen, with elastin exhibiting a limited turnover rate relative to collagen, (d) the phenotypic modulation of VSMCs toward more synthetic subpopulations and/or apoptosis of VSMCs, and (e) dysfunction in anti-inflammatory signaling pathways, such as the NO signaling pathway[11,12,136,137].

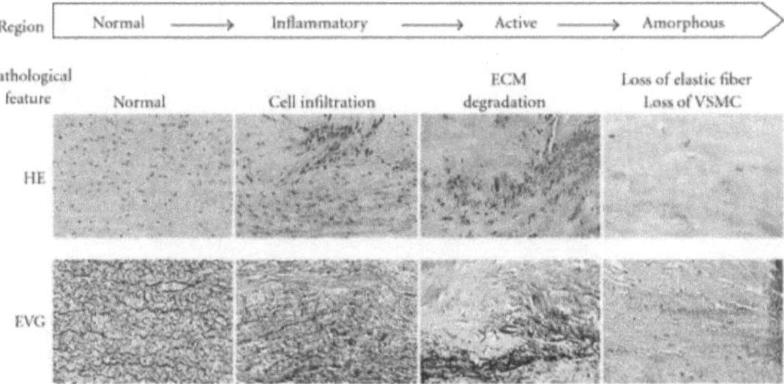

Figure 15: Histopathology of human AAAs reveals regional heterogeneity across three distinct zones (Inflammatory, Active, Amorphous), representing various stages of AAA progression, from early development to advanced phases[138]

Histological analysis of cross-sectional images from human AAAs reveals clear evidence of inflammatory and immune cell infiltration, including macrophages, neutrophils, mast cells, T and B lymphocytes, in both the medial and adventitial layers of

the aorta **(Figure 15)**[61,138–140]. These infiltrating cells are potent producers of cytokines and

chemokines, capable of directly influencing their own function as well as that of VSMCs.

Epidemiological studies have further confirmed these findings, showing a correlation

between elevated white blood cell (WBC) counts and ultrasound-based AAA detection.

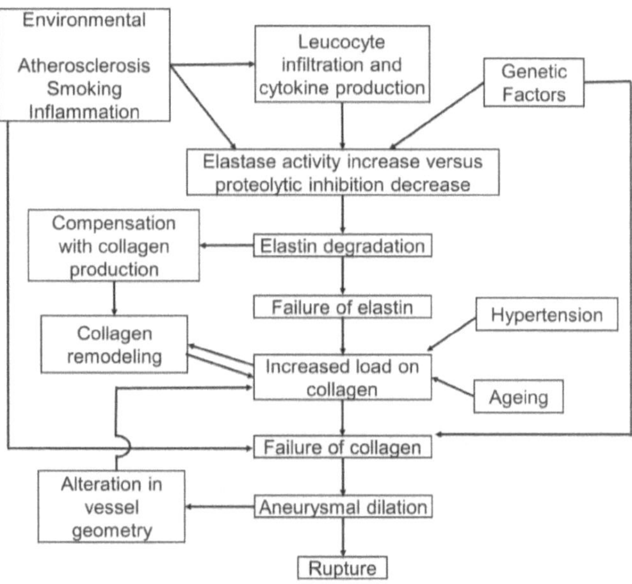

Figure 16: Block diagram showing the disease etiology of AAAs[137]

Upon activation by inflammatory cytokines, infiltrating immune cells release

numerous zinc-dependent endopeptidases, particularly MMPs, notably MMP2 and MMP9,

which have the potential to damage the fibrous extracellular matrix (ECM) proteins[140–142].

VSMCs also contribute to this process by producing both MMP2 and MMP9 in the aortal wall, resulting in a significant overexpression of total MMPs in AAA tissues and ultimately leading to elastic matrix degradation as shown by the active region. This inflammatory response represents the initial step in AAA formation and is strongly influenced by chronic stimuli such as hypertension, smoking, vasculitis, and the presence of preexisting plaques or atherosclerosis. The progression of AAA is illustrated in the accompanying flowchart (**Figure 16**).

The chronic overexpression of MMPs in the aorta shifts their balance towards generating a more proteolytic milieu and accelerated breakdown of both elastic and collagen fibers. While adult and diseased vascular cells can regenerate collagen quite readily and robustly, the ability to regenerate elastic fibers is very limited in adulthood and particularly in diseased scenarios. In compensation for the loss of elastic matrix, VSMCs increase collagen production, ultimately leading to loss of vessel elasticity and transient vessel stiffening prior to further weakening and rupture.

The degradation of the elastic matrix also generates elastin-degraded peptides (EDP), or elastokines, as mentioned earlier, which are bioactive and can amplify the inflammatory process[143]. This chronic degradation process, driven by factors like cytokines and EDPs, leads to an excessive accumulation of collagen compared to elastic, making the artery thinner, stiffer, and less compliant. Furthermore, increased forces on the weakened aortic wall trigger stress-activated mechanisms that stimulate more collagen production by VSMCs, attempting to stabilize AAA progression for a limited period (typically 5 to 7 years) before ultimately failing and leading to rupture.

Conversely, EDPs and inflammatory cytokines are also responsible for the apoptotic death of VSMCs, further contributing to vascular cell degradation[100,143]. Despite collagen having a good turnover rate, the compensatory mechanism of collagen production eventually halts at a critical point. Consequently, cells can no longer produce collagen, and the overexpressed MMPs continue to increase matrix degradation of both elastin and collagen. This imbalance in collagen synthesis and breakdown increases wall stress and the susceptibility of the aorta to fatal rupture. Furthermore, the intricate interplay between coagulation and inflammation, marked by the infiltration of leukocytes and cytokine production, culminates in thrombus formation, a common occurrence in AAAs[144]. As the aorta wall expands, the thrombus disrupts proper EC function, particularly their regulation of NO, an essential signaling molecule[145,146].

Endothelial cells play a pivotal role in synthesizing, metabolizing, and releasing various substances crucial for the regulation of vascular tone, blood pressure, coagulation cascades, fibrinolysis, inflammation, and reactive oxygen species (ROS) and reactive nitrogen species (RNS) involved in protein and lipid oxidation and nitrosylation[146]. Among these substances, NO plays a central role due to its regulation of anti-inflammatory, antiplatelet, antiproliferative, and antimigration processes in the aorta wall that contribute to maintaining tissue homeostasis. Dysfunctional NO signaling disrupts the delicate balance of vascular physiology, triggering inflammatory responses and exacerbating proteolytic degradation of the elastic matrix[146,147]. ROS and RNS are pivotal players in stimulating the degradation of the elastic matrix in AAAs. Excess ROS/RNS can activate MMPs, induce proinflammatory genes, and promote apoptosis, all of which are key characteristics of AAAs[148].

2.3.5   Chronic Inflammation and Immune Response in AAAs

The immune system is an intricate network comprising various immune cells, molecules, and pathways that regulate the body's overall equilibrium. The immune system is typically categorized into two components: innate immunity, which acts as the initial defense against pathogens, and adaptive immunity, developing later with the ability to demonstrate immunological memory[61,135]. When an injury stimulus is triggered, which may result from factors such as smoking, hypertension, vascular aging, or internal vascular diseases like thrombosis and atherosclerosis, it leads to chronic expression of specific enzymes, particularly MMP2 and MMP9[144]. These enzymes degrade the elastic matrix within the aortic wall. As a consequence of this degradation, fragments of elastin and collagen are formed, which act as primary attractants for infiltrating immune cells. This initiates an innate immune response aimed at compensating for the damage and restoring balance. However, in the context of AAAs, an inadequate equilibrium between inflammation and anti-inflammation prevails, contributing to aneurysm development and progression. The chronic inflammatory response is distributed transmurally, with the main site for infiltrating cells being the media and adventitia of the aortic wall. Predominantly, T lymphocytes and macrophages are the key infiltrating immune cells, with some presence of neutrophils and mast cells. Among the infiltrating lymphocytes, cluster of differentiation 4-positive (CD4$^+$) T lymphocytes are most abundant[61,138]. In human AAAs, high levels of interferon gamma (IFN-γ) are expressed which are often expressed by T-lymphocytes. Notably, the deficiency of both CD4 and IFN-γ has been shown to prevent cacl2-induced aneurysm[149]. Furthermore, IFN-γ significantly contributes to the activation of macrophages and stimulates the production of various pro-inflammatory cytokines, including IL-1β, IL-12, and IL-23, all of which are implicated in AAA growth[67]. Furthermore, the initial injury recruits pro-inflammatory M1 macrophages to sustain the ongoing inflammation, with the potential to transition to anti-inflammatory M2 macrophages that promote tissue repair through the production of anti-inflammatory cytokines like IL-10 and TGF-β[150]. Additionally, aside from T lymphocytes, both neutrophils and mast cells have the capacity to produce a wide range of inflammatory cytokines and chemokines, including IL-1, IL-3, IL-4, IL-5, Il-6, TNF-α, and IFN-γ, as well as various proteases like chymase, tryptase, and cathepsins[67,135]. Collectively, these immune responses activate MMPs, contributing to the development and progression of AAAs.

2.4 Role of Intracellular Signal Transduction Pathways in AAAs

Numerous intracellular signaling pathways play crucial roles in the formation and progression of AAAs. Many of these pathways are initiated by cytokines and chemokines, with a particular emphasis on TGF-β, TNF-α, and IL-1β [62,66,67]. Inhibition of TGF-β or the removal of the SMAD3 gene systemically has been observed to enhance the development of Angiotensin II and CaCl$_2$-induced AAAs. Activation of the SMAD signaling pathway subsequently leads to an increase in downstream MMP2 and MMP9 levels[151]. Furthermore, NOTCH 1 is another signaling mediator found in both human AAAs and Ang II-induced mouse models. Pharmacological inhibition of NOTCH 1 has been shown to mitigate AAAs by preventing macrophage infiltration and downregulating inflammation-induced proteolytic expressions[63].

The mitogen-activated protein kinases (MAPK) pathways represent another important signaling pathway involved in AAAs **(Figure 17)**. MAPKs represent highly conserved signaling proteins that play pivotal roles across a wide spectrum of organisms, spanning from yeast to humans[152]. They constitute a fundamental component of phosphorylation cascades, encompassing MAPK kinase kinase (MAPKKK), which phosphorylates and activates MAPK kinase (MAPK), ultimately resulting in the activation of MAPK. These cascades respond to diverse extracellular stimuli, eliciting specific biological consequences and regulatory mechanisms. Within the MAPK family, c-Jun N-Terminal Kinase (JNK) and the extracellular signal-regulated kinases (ERKs) are activated primarily by cytokines (e.g. TNF-α, and IL-1β) and are crucial to the adverse molecular regulation of MMP secretion and vascular wall remodeling that are central to AAA pathophysiology[152].

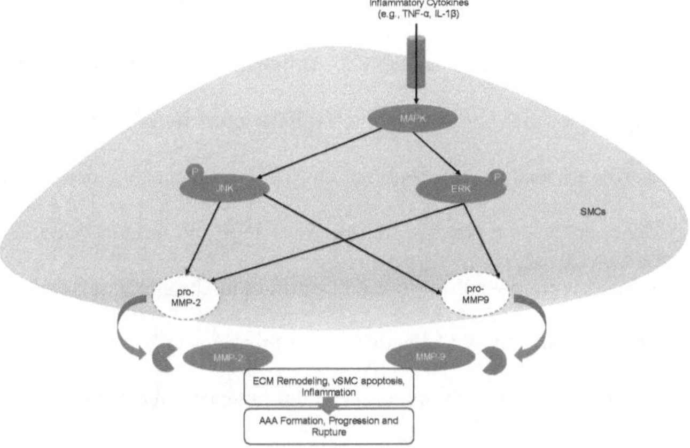

Figure 17: Exploration of MAPK signaling pathways and their pivotal role in regulating MMPs within vSMCs during AAAs. The diagram focuses on the activation of MAPK, specifically JNK and ERK pathways, shedding light on their contribution to the modulation of MMPs in the context of AAAs [153]

2.4.1 JNK signaling Pathway

JNK is categorized as a stress-activated protein kinase due to its activation in response to wide range of cellular stresses as well as to inflammatory mediators[154]. This pathway interacts with and phosphorylates the DNA binding protein c-Jun, enhancing transcriptional activities within cells. The regulation of JNK is intricate, influenced by numerous MAPKKK proteins. In animals with arterial injuries, MAPKs, including JNK, are rapidly and transiently activated, exerting control over various VSMC processes[155]. Intriguingly, JNK has been found in abundance within AAAs, positively influencing MMP expression[156]. Multiple studies propose JNK as a potential AAA target, as its inhibition not only suppresses degradation pathways but also facilitates the restoration of biosynthetic pathways for ECM repair[157]. The specificity of JNK signaling likely arises from crosstalk among different MAPKKKs, close interactions with upstream and downstream components, and functional overlap between JNK isoforms. JNK comprises three isoforms: JNK1, JNK2, and JNK3, with JNK1 and JNK2 being ubiquitously expressed throughout various bodily systems, exhibiting functional redundancy. In contrast, JNK3 is primarily associated with neuronal and cardiovascular functions. Additionally, emerging evidence suggests a possible link between JNK and inflammation, as evidenced by JNK-dependent immune cell infiltration, resulting in chronic upregulation of proinflammatory cytokine production[158]. Collectively, these findings indicate that targeted inhibition of JNK may reduce chronic inflammation and thus attenuate AAA pathogenesis.

2.4.2 ERK Signaling Pathway

The ERK signaling pathway responds to various extracellular factors, including growth factors, hormones, and cellular stresses, orchestrating cellular processes. Activation of this pathway commences with the activation of cell membrane receptors such as Tyrosine kinase receptors (RTKs), G protein-coupled receptors (GPCRs), and ion channels[159]. These receptors transduce signals, initiating the activation of Ras proteins in the cell membrane. This triggers a series of downstream events, involving proteins and transcription factors that regulate gene and protein expression, subsequently governing cellular proliferation, migration, and apoptosis. ERK comprises two isoforms, ERK1 and ERK2, which exhibit functional redundancy but possess a broad functional scope[160]. Due to their wide substrate recognition, activated ERKs can phosphorylate numerous regulatory proteins located in both the cytoplasm and nucleus. In the context of AAAs, the ERK pathway is known to play a well-defined role in disease pathogenesis. The expression of ERK1 and ERK2 is upregulated in AAA patients. Knockdown of ERK, specifically ERK1 -/- in male C57BL/6 mice, has been shown to prevent AAA formation, leading to a decrease in MMP2 and MMP9[16]. ERK also contributes to the recruitment of neutrophils and other inflammatory cells that release cytokines. Notably, inflammatory cytokines such as IL-1β and TNF-α positively correlate with the expression of ERK, particularly phosphorylated ERK (pERK), and are associated with increased MMP expression in AAAs[153].

2.5 Nitric Oxide (NO)

Nitric oxide (NO) is a versatile signaling molecule with a rich history in biology, dating back to its discovery in the late 18th century. Its profound importance in biological systems was underscored by the Nobel Prize in Physiology and Medicine awarded in 1998 to Furchgott, Ignarro, and Murad for their pioneering work in establishing NO as a key physiological signaling agent[161]. NO's multifaceted actions, ranging from vasodilation to anti-inflammatory properties, have profound implications in understanding cardiovascular physiology and pathology.

2.5.1   Nitric Oxide in human physiology

NO is a diatomic, nonpolar molecule characterized by its stability and short biological half-life, lasting 2-6 seconds[46]. In the cardiovascular system, ECs are the primary producers of NO, through the enzymatic conversion of L-arginine by nitric oxide synthase (NOS). Notably, there are distinct isoforms of NOS, including endothelial NOS (eNOS), inducible NOS (iNOS), and neuronal NOS (nNOS). iNOS and nNOS are soluble enzymes located in the cytosol, contributing to neuro-signaling and immune defense[162]. In contrast, eNOS primarily associates with cell membranes, where it plays a pivotal role in regulating vascular function and platelet aggregation. In the context of platelet aggregation, which often initiates with inflammation in the endothelium, eNOS promotes NO production[163]. NO, in turn, activates soluble guanylate cyclase (sGC), leading to the conversion of guanosine triphosphate into cyclic guanosine monophosphate (cGMP). This process controls vasodilation and inhibits coagulation, with NO also suppressing the thromboxane A2 (TXA2) receptor to prevent platelet aggregation and inhibit thrombosis[164]. NO binds to few of the deoxygenated heme molecules in the oxygenated RBCs and through oxidation of β-globin Cys-93, allows efficient delivery of NO to promote vasodilation of the hypoxic tissues[163]. NO also regulates cardiac relaxation and modulates the heart. The regulatory roles of NO are summarized in **Figure 17**.

In the healthy blood vessel wall, NO exerts a protective role by suppressing VSMC proliferation and migration. Activation of cGMP-dependent protein kinases, initiated by cGMP, is critically involved in the transcriptional regulation MMPs[165]. NO also influences

mitogen-activated protein kinase (MAPK) cascades, including JNK, p38-MAPK, and ERK

pathways, which subsequently modulate nuclear factor-kappa beta (NF-κβ) activation[165].

Increasing evidence suggests that NO inhibits leukocyte activation and adhesion, further

contributing to its anti-inflammatory effects[46]. Experiments in various cell types have

shown that NO donors or enhanced NO bioavailability within the tissue inhibits the mRNA

stabilizing factor HuR and thus mediates a rapid decay of cytokine-induced MMP9 mRNA

in a cGMP-dependent manner[166].

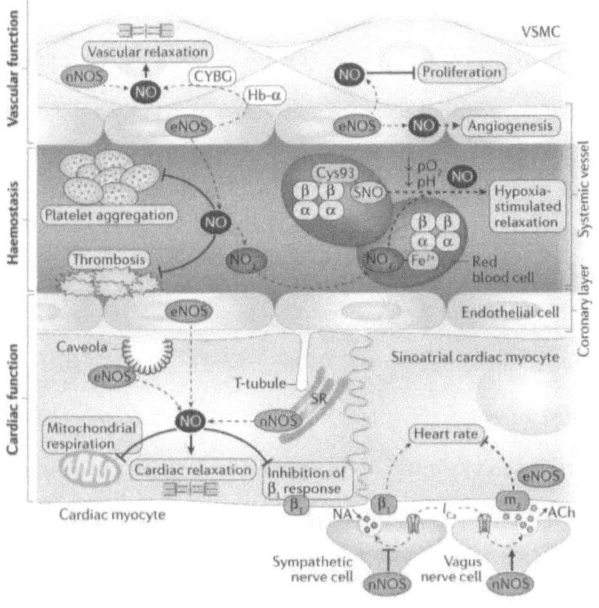

Figure 18: Schematic representation of the role of intrinsically produced NO in
cardiovascular health and cellular processes such as angiogenesis, thrombosis, platelet
aggregation and VSMC proliferation and migration[163]

In addition to this NO has also been shown to inhibit MMP2 expression in ECs[167]. In addition to its effects on mRNA stability, NO upregulates TIMP1, an MMP inhibitor, via the activation of latent TGF-β. This interaction is crucial in the ECM remodeling processes[168]. NO's influence extends to the signaling proteins JNK/SAPK. Having a cystine residue which is sensitive to thiol-modifying agents, NO downregulates JNK/SAPK via thiol-redox mechanism as NO being thiol-reactive molecule[169]. NO's further influences intracellular signaling proteins, including activated protein-1, NF-$\kappa\beta$, and Ras, which undergo s-nitrosylation, a modification mediated by NO[169,170]. This multifaceted role of NO underscores its significance in vascular physiology, where it impacts diverse processes critical for maintaining vascular health and homeostasis. As NO can mitigate many hallmarks of inflammation, NO may be able to provide selective effect in stabilizing/slowing the formation of AAAs.

2.5.2 Nitric Oxide donor drugs

NO donors are compounds designed to release NO in aqueous solutions, employing various chemical mechanisms. These donors are chosen based on the specific timescales required for their applications. However, the effectiveness of NO therapy is limited by the extremely short half-life of NO, its indiscriminate distribution, and challenges in reaching target tissues. To address these challenges, researchers have proposed several classes of NO donors and NO-related drugs, with four main categories: nitrites, metal nitrosyls, N-diazeniumdiolates (NONOates), and S-nitrosothiols **(Figure 19)** [171]. Among these, only nitrites and metal nitrosyls have received FDA approval.

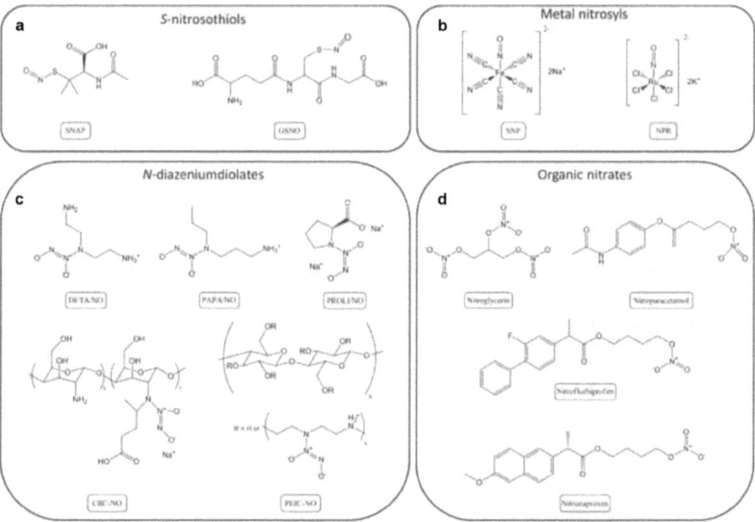

Figure 19: Categories of NO donor drugs, including a) S-nitrosothiols, b) Metal nitrosyls,
c) N-diazeniumdiolates, and d) Organic nitrates, highlighting diverse chemical
structures[171]

Nitrites, nitrates, and nitrosos do not directly release NO but rely on enzymatic
processes for reduction, ultimately producing NO[172]. NONOates decompose in aqueous
solutions through hydrolysis, and the rate of decomposition depends on factors like
molecular structure, temperature, and pH. However, they have not yet received FDA
approval for clinical use. S-nitrosothiols (RSNOs), such as GSNO, release NO through
homolytic cleavage, a process that can be influenced by factors like metallic ions, reducing
agents, enzymes, temperature, and pH[173]. Metal nitrosyls, on the other hand, are
photosensitive and sensitive to aqueous environments, allowing for controlled NO
delivery[174]. An example of metal nitrosyl is sodium nitroprusside (SNP) which has been

66

widely used clinically as a vasorelaxant. These diverse classes of NO donors offer valuable options for NO-based therapies, each with its own set of advantages and considerations.

2.5.3   Sodium Nitroprusside

Sodium nitroprusside (chemical formula $Na_2[FeIII(CN)5(NO)]$), is a nonferromagnetic compound. When in a solution, SNP can undergo reduction by cysteine and glutathione, leading to the formation of the paramagnetic $[FeII(CN)_5(NO)]^{3-}$ radical. This radical eventually undergoes spontaneous decay through the dissociation of trans-cyanide ligands, resulting in $[Fe(CN)_4NO]^{2-}$ radical. Further decomposition of SNP involves cyano-trans elimination, ultimately releasing NO[175]. SNP is recognized for its potent NO-releasing properties and falls under the category of metal nitrosyls. In the vascular system, SNP works by enhancing vascular capacitance and inducing coronary vasodilation[176]. It is widely employed as a medication for the management of conditions such as hypertension and heart failure. One of its key advantages is the sustained release of NO, making it a valuable component in our research efforts[177].

2.6   Oral drug delivery and limitations

Oral drug administration is the most widely accepted and commonly used method for treating both systemic and local gastrointestinal diseases. It offers several advantages, including controlled drug delivery, ease of administration, and feasibility. The extensive surface area within the gastrointestinal tract, along with its thick mucosal layer, enhances drug attachment and subsequent absorption[25]. The mucous layer also provides some degree of protection against shear stress from peristaltic movements and guards against degradation by gastric juices. The abundant presence of enterocytes in the human intestines facilitates drug absorption, occurring through various pathways: transcellular, paracellular, carrier-mediated transcellular, and facilitated transport[178].

Despite being the preferred method for drug delivery, oral administration of drugs faces several challenges due to barriers encountered in the gastrointestinal tract, circulatory system, and hepatic systems. Drugs must navigate three primary biological environments along the gut: the interior lumen, the mucosal layer, and the underlying tissue[25,178]. The acidic conditions of the stomach can potentially denature drugs and reduce their effectiveness. While pH-sensitive carriers (e.g., hydrogels) can encapsulate drugs to shield them from enzymatic degradation by lipases, trypsins, amylases, and peptidases in the stomach and intestines, achieving precise pH-dependent drug release may not always be practical, as it can affect drug availability at the target tissue[178]. Additionally, the gastrointestinal epithelium consists of a phospholipid bilayer that may permit the passage of lipophilic drugs or macromolecules while limiting the transit of hydrophilic drugs[25].

Due to these challenges, numerous drug delivery systems, specifically nanocarriers or nanoparticles (NPs), are currently under development to address the limitations imposed by the gastrointestinal tract. Researchers are also exploring alternative routes of administration to enhance drug delivery and efficacy.

2.7   Tissue-Localized Drug Delivery

Nanomedicine encompasses a wide array of nanoparticulate systems constructed from diverse materials, including synthetic polymers, inorganic compounds, metals, and lipids, all with the primary objective of serving as delivery vehicles for therapeutic agents. In recent years, significant strides have been made in the field of nanomedicine, particularly in material science, nanotechnology, and nanotherapeutics. These advancements have paved the way for the development of various drug-encapsulating NPs typically ranging in size from 1 nm to several hundred nanometers. However, their drug delivery capabilities can be influenced by various physiological factors, depending on the target tissue and application. These NPs are designed to safeguard drugs from premature degradation in the *in-vivo* environment, prevent drug leakage, enhance drug absorption by facilitating diffusion across epithelial barriers, modulate drug distribution profiles and pharmacokinetics, improve cellular uptake for localized effects, increase drug efficiency and efficacy, and finely regulate physiological responses as needed. However, it's crucial to note that not all NPs are suitable for drug delivery to animals and humans. Their suitability depends on factors such as biocompatibility, biodegradability, appropriate half-life and stability, and the absence of toxicity or inflammation-inducing properties.

2.7.1 Nanoparticles for Drug Delivery

Among the various types of materials used in formulating NPs, organic polymers stand out as the most extensively employed nanoparticulate system. This preference arises from their straightforward preparation, capacity for high-throughput formulation, biodegradability and accessibility to controlled polymer degradation through both chemical and enzymatic processes for sustained release, successful track record in drug delivery, and more[179]. Polymer-based NPs offer distinct advantages, allowing for the fine-tuning of solubility, drug release profiles, diffusivity, bioavailability, and immunogenicity[179,180]. Consequently, these modifications can result in reduced toxicity, fewer side effects, enhanced biodistribution, and an extended half-life of the drug in the bloodstream. These NPs can be tailored for site-specific targeting through surface functionalization or designed for controlled delivery at specific sites via direct administration. The formation of these NPs involves self-assembly in water and is engineered to surmount barriers such as opsonization or systemic clearance by the immune system[179]. Below is a list of the most used polymeric NPs shown in **Figure 20**.

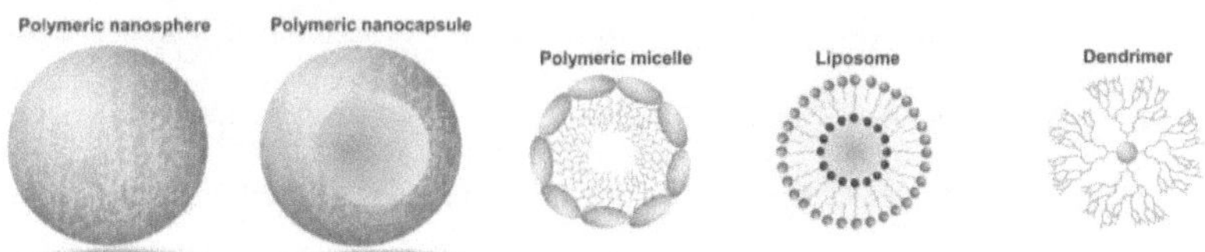

Figure 20: Showing different types of commonly used NPs[181]

2.7.1.1 Micelles

Polymeric micelles are nanostructures made of amphiphilic block of copolymers that self-assemble to form a NP with a void core for drug encapsulation[179]. They consist of two distinct regions with opposite affinities towards a given solvent. These core structures permit the assimilation of hydrophobic drugs resulting in increased stability and bioavailability whereas hydrophilic shell offer solubility in water and can stabilize the core. Polymeric micelles can be fabricated through two primary methods a) by solvent-based direct dissolution of a polymer formed by dialysis in a suitable solvent, b) by the precipitation of one block by introducing a solvent[179,182]. Loading drugs into these polymeric micelles can be achieved through various techniques. This includes direct dissolution of the drug within a copolymer by incorporating a pre-made drug solution in an aqueous medium into this copolymer. Alternatively, drug incorporation can be

70

accomplished through a solvent evaporation process, where both the drug and copolymer are dissolved using an organic solvent and subsequently evaporated. Another approach involves the dialysis process, in which both the drug and copolymer, dissolved in an organic solvent, are combined within a dialysis bag and subjected to dialysis[182]. Their hydrophilic shell restrains non-specific interaction with biological components[179,180]. These micelles are smaller in size (<100 nm) which allows normal distribution to avoid clearance through kidneys, instead permitting them to accumulate to a specific location due to enhanced permeability and retention (EPR) effect thereby increasing efficacy of the drug. However, one drawback with polymeric micelles is that they offer poor control over the release kinetic of the drug due to their sensitivity to structural changes which make them less effective in terms of stable long-term delivery vehicles.

2.7.1.2 Polymeric Nanoparticles

Polymeric NPs exist in two primary forms: nanospheres and nanocapsules. Nanocapsules possess hollow-core structures with aqueous hydrophilic cores, providing the space needed for encapsulating hydrophilic substances such as drugs, DNAs, and RNAs[181,183]. In contrast, nanospheres consist of solid polymer matrices with the capability to incorporate hydrophobic drugs. These NPs can be crafted using one or more polymers, lipids, polysaccharides, and proteins, often employing the nanoemulsion technique. They exhibit a constant rate of payload release, yet they can pose challenges regarding purification and stability during long-term storage.

2.7.1.3 Dendrimers

Dendrimers represent branched polymer complexes produced through highly controlled polymerization techniques. They are highky bifurcated, monodisperse, well-defined three-dimensional structures. Their fabrication process is meticulously regulated, allowing for precise control of size and shape. Dendrimers possess excellent solubility and exhibit non-immunogenic properties[181]. However, dendrimers face constraints in their clinical utilization primarily because of the presence of amine groups, rendering them highly cationic and potentially toxic[179]. Loading drugs into dendrimers can be achieved through straightforward encapsulation, electrostatic interactions, or covalent conjugation. Drug release from dendrimers can occur through in vivo degradation of the covalent bond between the drug and dendrimer, facilitated by enzymatic activity, or through drug release triggered by variations in pH, temperature, or pressure differences[184].

2.7.1.4 Liposomes

Liposomes consist of natural lipids with both polar and non-polar components, facilitating self-assembly in aqueous environments. Liposomes offer several advantages, including FDA approval, high biocompatibility, ease of synthesis, and the ability to mitigate immunogenic responses[181]. Liposomes can be classified into four main types. Conventional liposomes consist of anionic, cationic, or neutral cholesterol and phospholipids, forming an aqueous core that can encapsulate both hydrophobic and hydrophilic drugs in the lipid bilayer and the aqueous space, respectively. PEGylated liposomes incorporate polyethylene glycol (PEG) on their surface to enhance stability and provide steric equilibrium. Ligand-targeted liposomes are designed by conjugating antibodies, carbohydrates, or peptides within the PEG chains, enabling specific targeting for drug delivery. Finally, theranostic liposomes amalgamate the characteristics of all previously mentioned liposome types and are frequently used for a variety of purposes, including targeted drug delivery, imaging, and therapeutic applications[179,185]. Regarding drug release, liposomes offer a controlled and leakage-free drug storage capability, thereby enhancing drug bioavailability within the therapeutic window at the appropriate rate and time[179]. However, conventional unmodified liposomes, when employed for drug delivery, can encounter opsonins, high-density lipoproteins (HDL), and low-density lipoproteins (LDL) within the in vivo body system. This interaction may lead to clearance or transportation of liposomes by HDL to the liver, resulting in their removal from the body. This limitation underscores the need for the development of modified liposomes, such as PEGylated liposomes, which possess stealth properties, enabling them to evade interactions with opsonins and HDL, and thus extending their potential applications[29,179,185]. Further details on liposomes are explored in section 2.7.2.

2.7.2 Liposomes or Lipid Nanoparticles (LNPs)

Liposomes or lipid nanoparticles (LNPs) are self-assembling nanoparticles characterized by their spherical structure, composed of lipid bilayers that encapsulate a portion of the surrounding solvent within their interior. These LNPs vary in size, ranging from 20 nm to several micrometers, and can feature one of several concentric membranes. Their structure and intrinsic diameter (d) categorize LNPs into different types, including multilamellar vesicles (MLV; d > 500 nm), which contain multiple concentric lipid bilayers within one LNP; small unilamellar vesicles (SUV; d < 100 nm) with a single layer; large

unilamellar vesicles (LUV; 100 ≤ d ≥ 1000 nm) with a single layer; and multivesicular

vesicles (MVV; d > 100 nm) containing multiple non-concentric liposomes (**Figure 21**)[186].

The versatile design and engineering options available for LNPs render them invaluable

tools across a wide spectrum of biomedical applications.

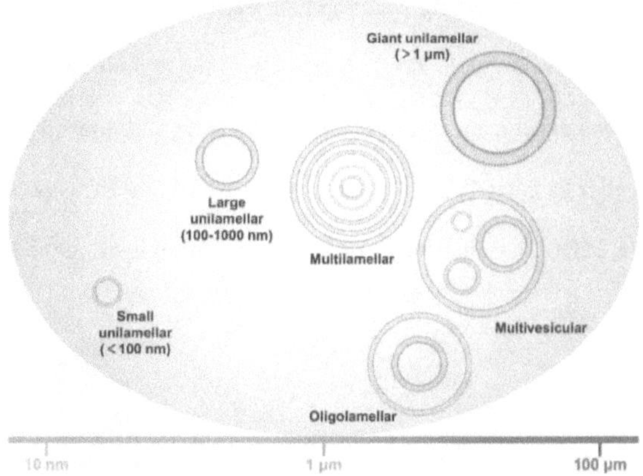

Figure 21: Categorization of liposomes based on vesicle diameter and lamellarity. Small
unilamellar vesicles (SUVs) measure less than 100 nm, while large unilamellar vesicles
(LUVs) fall within the range of 100 to 1000 nm. Giant unilamellar vesicles (GUVs)
surpass the 1 µm threshold. Oligolamellar vesicles (OLVs) share similarities with
multilamellar vesicles (MLVs), exhibiting concentric bilayers. Multivesicular vesicles
(MVVs) feature multiple non-concentric liposomes within the structure[186]

2.7.2.1 LNP Preparation Techniques

2.7.2.1.1 Thin-Film Hydration Method

This method stands as one of the oldest, most common, and simplest means of creating

LNPs[187,188]. The process initiates by mixing selected phospholipid components in an

organic solvent (e.g., chloroform, ethanol, dichloromethane, etc.) within a flask (**see**

74

Figure 22A). Subsequently, the mixture undergoes a rotary evaporation process at a temperature ranging from 45 to 60 °C, facilitating the evaporation of the organic solvent and leaving behind a thin film on the inner surface of the flask **(Figure 22B)**. Any residual organic solvent may be further eliminated using dry nitrogen, argon, or a basic vacuum desiccator. Once the solvent has been thoroughly removed, the thin film is then hydrated with a solution containing water and the desired drug, a process that takes approximately 1 to 2 hours **(Figure 22C)**. Typically, this technique results in the formation of multilamellar vehicles **(Figure 22D)**, which can subsequently be transformed into small unilamellar vesicles (SUVs) of uniform size through extrusion using a specialized device **(Figure 22E)**. The final stages of LNP preparation involve their purification and physical characterization.

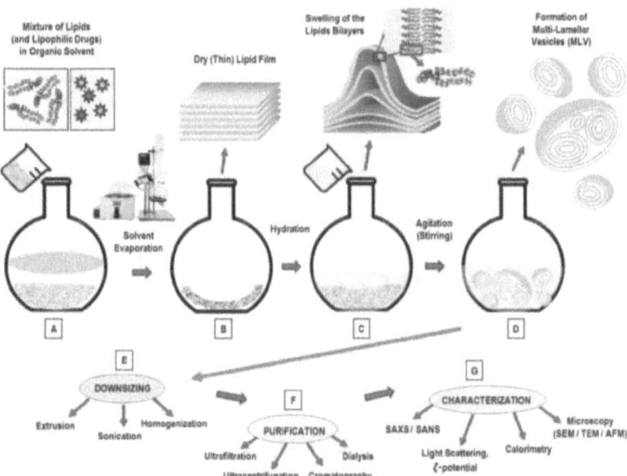

Figure 22: Illustration of the thin film hydration technique, encompassing A) lipid mixing, and organic solvent evaporation, B) thin film creation, C) hydration with an aqueous solution, and D) agitation to induce liposome formation. Following liposome generation, additional steps can be undertaken for E) size control, F) purification, and G) characterization[188]

2.7.2.1.2 Detergent Removal Method

In this approach, a blend of lipids is hydrated by employing detergents like sodium cholate, Triton X-100, sodium deoxycholate, among others. When these components are combined, detergents associate with the phospholipids, facilitating their self-assembly. This process leads to the creation of micelles, as the detergent shields the hydrophobic segments from direct interaction with the aqueous phase. Subsequently, the detergent is removed by dialysis, chromatography or adsorption onto hydrophobic beads or dilution to obtain unilamellar vesicles[188,189].

2.7.2.1.3 Solvent Injection Method

This is accomplished by dissolving lipids in ethanol or ether, both of which are organic solvents[189]. The lipid solution is then injected into the aqueous phase. In the ethanol injection method, phospholipids are rapidly introduced into preheated water, promoting the self-assembly of lipids. This process facilitates the fusion of self-assembled lipid bilayers to create vesicles. On the other hand, in the ether injection method, lipids are dissolved in ether and slowly injected into an aqueous phase at temperatures ranging from 55 to 65 °Celsius. The gradual removal of the organic solvent under reduced pressure results in the formation of large unilamellar vesicles (LUVs). This technique yields LNPs with a size ranging from 60 to 200 nm, indicating a favorable polydispersity index[188].

2.7.2.1.4 Reverse-phase evaporation method

In this method, lipids are dissolved in a mixture of organic solvents at specific volume ratios, such as 1:1 for ether/chloroform or 2:1 for chloroform/methanol[188]. The aqueous phase is then introduced into this mixture, leading to the self-arrangement of lipids, creating a water-in-oil microemulsion[189]. This microemulsion can be homogenized using sonication techniques to facilitate the uniform formation of LNPs. Subsequently, the mixture undergoes rotary evaporation to remove the organic solvent, resulting in the formation of a viscous, gel-like structure that eventually collapses to yield liposomes[188].

2.7.2.2 Post Processing for precise control of LNP Size

Depending on the specific application, precise control over the size, polydispersity index, lamellarity, and homogeneity of LNPs is often required. To achieve this level of control, post-processing techniques are employed, and three main methods are commonly used, each offering control over various parameters as explained below.

2.7.2.2.1 Sonication

This method involves the application of high-energy ultrasound, which generates localized warming in the lipid particle-containing solution, resulting in the formation of small unilamellar vesicles (SUVs). However, this technique has some drawbacks, including potential contamination from metal wear at the tip, increased heat which might lead to de-esterification, and reduced encapsulation efficiency of lipids for drugs.

2.7.2.2.2 Extrusion

Extrusion is employed to pass a hydrated lipid solution through membranes containing small pores. Repeated back-and-forth extrusion forces the NPs through these pores, effectively filtering the LNPs by size and ensuring a homogeneous distribution[187]. While this technique is highly reproducible and widely accepted, it can lead to significant liquid loss if not executed carefully, thus reducing the overall yield[188].

2.7.2.2.3 High-Pressure Homogenization

In this method, the lipid suspension is continuously injected through an orifice at high pressure, where it collides with a stainless-steel wall, resulting in the formation ofLNPs. Shear forces, turbulence, and cavitation play pivotal roles in LNP formation. However, this technique tends to yield LNPs with a broader size distribution, making it less suitable for achieving smaller, homogeneous LNPs.

2.7.2.3 Drug Loading in LNPs

High drug loading is highly desirable as it serves several purposes, such as minimizing the need for excipients, achieving the desired concentration of therapeutic agents, reducing the volume of the dose, and shortening dosing time. Drug loading in LNPs can be achieved through passive loading, active loading, or drug-lipid conjugation.

Passive loading involves entrapping hydrophilic drugs within the core of LNPs during the formation of the lipid bilayer when the LNPs are hydrated[29,189]. During this process, hydrophobic drugs are encapsulated within the hydrophobic region formed between the lipid bilayers. Most commonly, encapsulation is achieved through covalent, ionic, electrostatic, non-covalent, or steric interactions between the drug and the lipid. However, passive loading may sometimes lead to lipid bilayer destabilization, high drug-to-lipid ratios, rapid or burst drug release, resulting in low encapsulation efficiency, which may necessitate an additional step for residual drug removal.

Active loading creates a gradient between the LNP core and the drug in the solution. This gradient can be based on factors such as pH differences or ionic variances across the lipid bilayer[29]. Active loading primarily relies on the solubility of the drug in the solution and the presence of ions when the drug decomposes. This technique can be employed with various LNP formulation methods and generally results in greater encapsulation and loading efficiency.

An alternative approach to drug loading involves covalently linking drug molecules to lipids using a linker molecule forming a drug-lipid conjugation[190].

2.7.2.4 LNPs for the Delivery of Therapeutic Agents

Since gaining FDA approval in 1995, LNP formulation has been extensively employed as a drug delivery system for the localized treatment of various diseases, including cancer, infections, pain management, hepatitis A, and influenza[29,191]. Numerous liposome-based drugs designed for human use are administered through various routes such as intravenous, intramuscular, intrathecal injection, epidural, local infiltration, or oral inhalation[191]. In the cardiovascular domain, LNPs have been utilized for diagnostic and therapeutic purposes. *Ex-vivo* studies on Langendorff-isolated rat hearts have demonstrated cardioprotective effects when LNPs loaded with ATP were administered via intracoronary infusion[192].

Moreover, liposome-plasmid DNA complexes modified with the cell-penetrating transactivating transcriptional activator peptide (TATp) in rats with experimental myocardial infarction showed enhanced liposome accumulation in the ischemic zone with improved transfection within cardiomyocytes[193]. LNPs have also been investigated for delivering thrombolytic agents in a rabbit jugular vein thrombosis model, exhibiting significantly enhanced thrombolytic efficiency compared to blank LNPs. In a rabbit model of atherosclerosis, LNP formulation of glucocorticoids, designed for simultaneous monitoring and delivery of an anti-inflammatory drug, displayed notable anti-inflammatory effects within two days of intravenous injection, highlighting their potential as an advanced drug delivery tool[194].

In conclusion, LNPs stand out as a superior drug delivery system with their multifaceted applications and demonstrated efficacy in localized disease treatment. Their versatility is underscored by FDA approval for various therapeutic areas, ranging from cancer to infections and cardiovascular diseases. LNPs offer a range of administration routes, providing flexibility in tailoring treatment strategies to specific patient needs. Studies exploring their use in cardiovascular applications, such as cardioprotective effects and targeted drug delivery in ischemic zones, showcase their potential in advancing cardiac care. LNPs also exhibit promise in thrombolytic therapy and atherosclerosis treatment, all of which are often associated with AAAs, indicating their versatility in addressing complex medical conditions[144]. With ongoing advancements and research, LNPs emerge as a forefront tool for enhanced drug delivery, offering improved precision, efficacy, and potential for personalized therapeutic interventions.

CHAPTER III: Sodium Nitroprusside-Stimulation of Elastic Matrix Regeneration by Aneurysmal Smooth Muscle Cells

3.1 Introduction

As discussed in the previous chapter, AAAs are naturally irreversible expansions of the aortal wall that result from the enzymatic degradation of elastic fibers by chronically overexpressed MMPs. The pathophysiology of AAAs is multifaceted, involving factors such as the infiltration of leukocytes, the production of pro-inflammatory cytokines, apoptosis of vascular smooth muscle cells, diminished NO signaling, endothelial dysfunction, and the phenotypic transition of vascular smooth muscle cells between contractile and synthetic phenotypes[11,12]. Currently, there are no established therapies to reverse AAA pathophysiology, particularly in restoring elastic matrix homeostasis, which would be essential to slow or halt the growth of small (<5 cm diameter) AAAs before they reach a larger, pre-rupture stage necessitating risky surgical intervention. The availability of drug-based regenerative matrix therapies could significantly impact the management of this condition.

As previously mentioned, in inflamed vascular tissues, NO has shown to inhibit MAPKs such as JNK, ERKs, and p38, all of which are significantly upregulated in AAAs[155,156] Such inhibition can subsequently attenuate the downstream expression of MMPs, to reduce proteolytic disruption and loss of the structural ECM in the vessel wall. Previous research in our laboratory has indicated that the attenuation of JNK significantly enhances the neoassembly of elastic fibers and reduces MMP activity in aneurysmal

SMCs[195]. Given the evidence that endogenously-generated NO downregulates MMPs and inhibits JNK phosphorylation and activation[21], this study aims to investigate whether exposing primary human aneurysmal SMCs (aHASMCs) to a NO donor drug, sodium nitroprusside (SNP), can be a valuable therapeutic approach for restoring ECM homeostasis, particularly in terms of reinstating intact and crosslinked elastic fiber structures, which does not naturally occur.

3.2   Materials and Methods

3.2.1   Isolation and Culture of aHASMCs From Human AAA Tissue Biopsies

AAA tissues were obtained from patients undergoing open surgical repair of large abdominal aortic aneurysms at a pre-rupture stage, under the auspices of an IRB protocol at the Cleveland Clinic. Primary aHASMCs were isolated and characterized as previously described[196]. First, the intimal layer comprised of endothelial cells was scraped off from the AAA tissue, and the medial layer was separated from the underlying adventitial layer and adipose tissue. Then, the sliced tissue was further cut into pieces of roughly 5 mm^2 and subjected to a two-step enzymatic digestion process in Dulbecco's modified Eagle medium and Ham's F-12 medium (DMEM/F12; Thermo Fisher Scientific, Waltham, MA), first with 125 U/mg collagenase type I (Worthington Biochemicals, Lakewood, NJ) for 20 min at 37 °C, and then with 3 U/mg elastase (Worthington Biochemicals) for 1 h in a temperature-controlled shaker at 37 °C . The digestates were then centrifuged (1245 rpm, 10 min) and transferred to a 10-cm^2 culture dish (6-well plate). The culture surface of each well was scratched with a sterile scalpel blade to create grooves for cell attachment.

Primary aHASMCs, derived by outgrowth of the digestates, were cultured for 14 to 21 days in DMEM/F12 medium supplemented with 20% v/v fetal bovine serum (FBS; Gibco, Waltham, MA) and 1% v/v penicillin-streptomycin (PenStrep; Thermo Fisher Scientific, Waltham, MA) and then transferred to a T-25 flask for further propagation. aHASMCs from passages 2 to 6 were used for experiments.

3.2.2   Determining IC50 Value of SNPs for Viability of aHASMCs

The IC50 (50% inhibitory concentration of the drug on cell survival) of SNP (Sigma, Burlington, MA) was assessed using a 3-(4,5-dimethylthiazol-2-yl)-2,5-diphenyl tetrazolium bromide (MTT) assay (Abcam, Waltham, MA). Two days post-seeding, aHASMCs cultures (3×10^4 cells/well, 6-well plates, n = 3), were treated with SNP (100 pM – 10 mM) reconstituted in DMEM/F12 medium containing 1% v/v Pen-Strep and 2% v/v FBS for the 24 h; control cultures received no SNP. MTT reagent (0.5 mg/mL in PBS) was then added to each well and incubated for 3 h to allow the formation of a blue crystalline formazan product. The formazan was solubilized using 300 μL of dimethyl sulfoxide (DMSO), and 200 μL of each sample was taken in a 96-well plate, and absorbance was measured at a wavelength of 570 nm.

3.2.3   Cytokine-Injury Cell Culture Model

In AAAs, infiltrating immune cells continuously secrete pro-inflammatory cytokines, contributing to the proteolytic damage of the elastic matrix within the AAA wall by MMPs[62]. Therefore, cytokine-injury (cytokine-exposed) cell culture model was established in this study to closely mimic the inflammatory milieu of AAAs. In this experiment, aHASMCs were seeded in chamber slides for 48 h and serum-starved in DMEM/F12 medium containing 2% v/v FBS for 3 h. Immediately after serum starving, aHASMC cultures were treated with a cocktail of 10 ng/mL of tumor necrosis factor-alpha (TNFα; Thermo Fisher Scientific) and 10 ng/mL of interleukin-1 beta (IL-1β; R&D systems, Minneapolis, MN) for various time points (0 min, 30 min, 1 h, 2 h, 3 h, 24 h) to determine the optimal time for disease exaggeration as a function of upregulated MMP2 expression. MMP2 expression in each culture was visualized using immunofluorescence (IF) imaging with an Olympus IX51 fluorescence microscope (Olympus America, Center Valley, PA) as described in our experimental design section below.

3.2.4 Design of Cell Culture Experiments

For cell culture experiments, aHASMCs were seeded at a density of $3\times10^4 - 5\times10^4$ cells per well in a 6-well (A = 9.6 cm^2) or 15×10^3 cells per well in 12-well plate (A = 3.85 cm^2) /2-well chamber slides (A = 4 cm^2) and cultured in DMEM/F12 containing 10% v/v FBS for 7 days. On day 7, the cells were serum-starved in DMEM/F12 containing 2% v/v FBS for 3 h, followed by 3 h of cytokine treatment with a cocktail of TNFα (10 ng/mL) and IL-1β (10 ng/mL). This was followed by treating the cells with various doses of SNP (see above) for 7 days for gene and protein studies (or 14 days for elastic matrix quantification). The treatment was done every day by replenishing the DMEM/F12 media with a freshly prepared medium containing SNP in each of the culture wells. Control wells received media change each day without SNP treatment. Gene expression analysis was done using RT-PCR and qPCR SMC biology array, whereas protein expression was quantified using western blot, immunofluorescence, MAPK array, and biochemical assays for elastin, collagen, and DNA quantification. The overall experimental design is shown in

Figure 23.

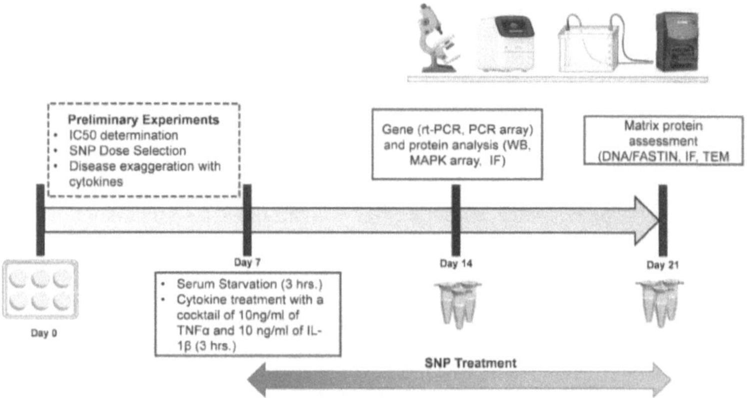

Figure 23: Schematics of *in vitro* experimental setup and timeline. From the
preliminary testing, the IC50 of SNP was determined, and further dosages were selected
based on the IC50 value. For disease exaggeration, the effect of incubation times with
inflammatory cytokines (TNFα: 10 ng/mL, IL1β: 10 ng/mL) on aHASMCs was verified
as a function of MMP2 expression at each time point. All protein and gene expression
studies involved 3 h of serum starving and 3 h of cytokine treatment on day 7, followed
by immediate SNP treatment in freshly prepared DMEM F-12 for 7 or 14 more days.
This figure was generated using images modified from Servier Medical Art, licensed
under a Creative Commons Attribution 3.0 license

3.2.5 Real-Time Polymerase Chain Reaction (RT-PCR)

Relative levels of gene expression between cases were determined by real-time PCR.

The total mRNA for this experiment (n = 6) was extracted after two weeks of culture using

the RNeasy mini kit (Qiagen, Valencia, CA) as per the manufacturer's instructions. The

total mRNA concentration was determined by Nanodrop 2000 spectrophotometer (Thermo

Fisher Scientific, Wilmington, DE). mRNA (200 ng) was reverse transcribed to cDNA

Table 5: Summary of SMC genes, their corresponding proteins, and their roles in elastic matrix homeostasis/SMC phenotype regulation[64,197]

Gene Nomenclature	Corresponding Protein	Role in Elastic Matrix Homeostasis
MYH11	Smooth muscle myosin heavy chain 11	Contractile apparatus protein, regulates SMC contraction and relaxation
ACTA2	Smooth muscle actin alpha 2	
DES	Desmin (Intermediate filament-class III)	Maintenance of structural and mechanical integrity of contractile apparatus
CNN	Calponin	Late-stage SMC marker of differentiated contractile phenotypes, colocalizes with actin filaments, regulates actin-myosin interaction
SMTN	Smoothelin	
MMP2 and *MMP9*	Matrix Metalloproteases 2 and 9	Proteolytic enzymes, degrades elastic and collagen fibers
TIMP1, TIMP2, TIMP4	Tissue Inhibitors of matrix metalloproteases 1, 2 and 4	Inhibitor of MMPs
MAPK 1, MAPK 2	Extracellular signal-regulated kinase 2 (ERK 2) and 1 (ERK 1) respectively	Regulated by extracellular signals, sacts as a critical intermediate in inflammatory response and proteases synthesis
MAPK 8, MAPK 9	c-Jun N-terminal kinase 1(JNK 1) and 2 (JNK 2) respectively	Stress activated protein kinase, acts as a critical intermediate in inflammatory response and proteases synthesis
ELN	Elastin	Core elastic fiber protein in the aorta, provide elastic recoil properties to the aorta wll, provides structural support
LOX	Lysyl oxidase	Crosslinks elastin to form matured elastic fibers
COLIA1, COLIIIA1	Collagen Type I alpha 1, Collagen Type III alpha 1 respectively	Core ECM fibrillar protein of the aorta, provides strength and load bearing properties

Table 6: List of primer sequences used for RT-PCR

Primer	Forward Sequence (5'-3')	Reverse Sequence (5'-3')
18s	TCA AGA ACG AAA GTC GGA GG	GGA CAT CTA AGG GCA TCA CA
MMP2	TTG ACG GTA AGG ACG GAC TC	ACT TGC AGT ACT CCC CAT CG
TIMP1	TAC TTC CAC AGG TCC CAC AA	ATT CCT CAC AGC CAA CAG TG
TIMP2	TAT AAC ACC CCA CCC CTG TT	AAG GAA TCC ACC TGC ATA GG
TIMP4	CTC TTC CCT CTG TGG TGT GA	TGT CCA GAG GCA CTC GTT AG
ERK1	ATT TGT GAT TTC GGC CTG GC	TCG GGC CTT CAT GTT GAT GA
ERK2	CAG TGG GAT GGA ATT GAA AG	AGC AGA AGG AAT GAG TGT GC
JNK1	GTG CAT TAT GGG AGA AAT GG	GTT CTG AGT CAG CTG GGA AA
JNK2	CTT CAT GAT GAC CCC TTA CG	AAT ATG GTC AGT GCC TTG GA
ELN	CAG TTG GTA CCC AAG CAC CT	AGG TGG CTA TTC CCA GTG TG
LOX	CAG AGG AGA GTG GCT GAA GG	CCA GGT AGC TGG GGT TTA CA
FBN1	CAC ACA ACT GTG GCA AAC AT	CCC ATG GTA TTC TTG CAG TC
FBLN4	GGA AAT GAA GTG CAT CAA CC	TAG GAG CCA GGC AAG TTA TG
FBLN5	CAT TGC AGT GAT ATG GAC GA	GAA GCC CCC TTG TAA ATT GT
COL1A1	TTC TGC TCC TTT CTC CAC AC	TCT TTG GCA GTC TGA GAA CC
COL3A1	AGC TAC GGC AAT CCT GAA CT	GGG CCT TCT TTA CAT TTC CA
ACTA	AGT TAC GAG TTG CCT GAT GG	GAG GTC CTT CCT GAT GTC AA
DES	CAG ACC TAC TCT GCC CTC AA	TAG AGC ACT TCA TGC TGC TG
MYH11	AGC CAG AGA CGA GAG GAC AT	ACG GTT CCT GGA ACA TCT C
SMTH	TGT GAC CAC AGT GAC ACT CC	AGA AGC TTG TTG ACC ACC TG
CNN	CTC CCA AGT GAC TGG ATT TG	ACT GAG GCC AGA GTG AGT TG

using the iScript cDNA synthesis kit (Bio-Rad, Hercules, CA) in a thermocycler as instructed by the manufacturer. The expression of SMC- specific genes was quantified

87

using SYBR® Green master mix and target-specific primers (RealtimePrimers; Elkins Park, PA) in Quantstudio® 3 (Applied Biosystems; Thermo Fisher Scientific). The relative gene expression of each target was determined by using the ΔΔCt method as explained by Livak *et al*[198]. Data were normalized to the endogenous reference gene (*18s*). The roles of the proteins whose gene expression was analyzed are specified in **Table 5**. **Table 6** lists the primers and their respective sequences used in this study.

3.2.6 Western Blot (WB) Analysis for ECM Homeostasis Proteins

The protein expression in each sample was assessed semi-quantitatively using WB analysis. aHASMCs were harvested in RIPA buffer (Thermo Fisher Scientific) containing 1% v/v Halt™ protease inhibitor and phosphatase inhibitor (Thermo Fisher Scientific). Total protein expression was determined using a colorimetric bicinchoninic acid (BCA) assay kit (Thermo Fisher Scientific). The protein samples (2 μg) mixed with the loading buffer and a reducing agent were loaded in 10% or 4 -12% NuPAGE™ Bis-Tris gels. SeeBlue® pre-stained ladder was used for molecular weight approximation. The gel was then subjected to sodium dodecyl sulfate-polyacrylamide gel electrophoresis (SDS-PAGE) (Thermo Fisher Scientific) and transferred to a nitrocellulose membrane using iBlot® Western Blotting System (Invitrogen). The transferred membranes were blocked, and incubated overnight with primary antibodies (**Table 7**), followed by secondary antibody incubation (with IRDye® 680LT goat-anti-rabbit secondary antibody in (1:15,000 dilutions) and IRDye® 800CW goat anti-mouse secondary antibody (1:20,000 dilution) as described in our published work[195,199].

Table 7: Details of primary antibodies used in western blot and immunofluorescence

Protein	WB dilution (v/v)	IF dilution (v/v)	Catalog no.	Source
MMP2	1:1000	1:200	ab92536	Abcam
TIMP1	1:1000	1:200	bs-0415R	Thermo Fisher Scientific
TIMP2	1:1000	1:200	ab180630	Abcam
TIMP4	1:1000	1:200	ab38987	Abcam
LOX	1:1000	1:50	ab31238	Abcam
JNK	1:1000	1:200	44-682G	Thermo Fisher Scientific
p-JNK	-	1:200	AF1205	R&D Systems
ERK	1:1000	1:200	9102S	Cell Signaling Technology
p-ERK	-	1:200	9101S	Cell Signaling Technology
FBN	1:1000	1:100	PA5-99225	Thermo Fisher Scientific
ELN	1:1000	1:100	ab217356	Abcam
β-actin	1:2000	NA	MAB8929	R&D Systems

3.2.7 Gelatin Zymography for MMP2 Activity

The enzyme activity of MMP2 was determined by gel zymography. Briefly, 2 µg of protein was loaded in each well alongside MMP2 standard. Then the gels were run in an electrophoresis unit at 125 V as discussed in our WB experiments. The gels were then renatured in 2.5% Triton-X-100, developed in the 1X Novex development buffer and stained with SimplyBlue SafeStain. The de-staining of the gels was done in DI water for 72 h. After de-staining, MMP2 bands on a dark background were quantified using ImageJ software.

3.2.8 PCR Array for SMC Biology-Focused Genes

For SMC biology-focused gene expression analysis of cultured aHASMCs, a human qPCR array kit (ScienceCell™ research laboratories, Carlsbad, CA) was used. Selected SNP doses (0 M, 100 nM) study was evaluated in comparing the gene expression profile of a total of 88 genes (no replicates during analysis) relevant to SMC biological function, contraction, phenotypic switching, and ECM synthesis. mRNA (35 ng) from our RT-PCR sample was pooled from each sample/per group (n = 6) to comprise a final concentration of 210 ng mRNA. The mRNA was then reverse transcribed to cDNA using the iScript cDNA synthesis kit. cDNA amplification was done in Quantstudio® 3 using KAPA SYBR fast qPCR master mix (2×) ROX low (Roche Sequencing and life sciences, Indianapolis, IN). Gene expression was analyzed using the ΔΔCt method. The data were normalized to the geometric mean of 5 different housekeeping genes (β-Actin, GAPDH, LDHA, NONO, PPIH) and presented as log2 fold change to determine the multiplicative factor of upregulation or downregulation of the target gene vs. control.

3.2.9   LIVE/DEAD™ Assay for Cell Viability

To assess the effect of SNP dose on aHASMC viability, a LIVE/DEAD™ viability/cytotoxicity kit (Thermo Fisher Scientific) was used. The SNP doses were 500 nM, 100 nM, and 1 μM. For this experiment, 15×10^3 cells/well were seeded in a 12-well plate and cultured for 7 days. Cells were then serum-starved, and cytokine treated as explained in our experimental design section. Following the cytokine treatment, cells were then treated with SNP for 24 h. Subsequently, the cells were stained with calcein-AM and ethidium homodimer-1, as per the manufacturer's instructions, to determine the percentage of viable and dead cells.

3.2.10 DNA Assay for Cell Proliferation

The effect of SNP dose on aHASMC proliferation over 21 days of culture was determined using a Hoechst-33248 dye-based fluorometric DNA assay as described earlier[200]. Briefly, in this dose escalation study, aHASMCs were seeded in 6-well plates (5×10^4 cells/well) and treated with SNP at doses of 100 nM, 250 nM, and 500 nM. The cells were cultured for 21 days, harvested using Pi Buffer (50 mM Na_2HPO_4, 2 mM EDTA, 0.3 mM NaN_3), and sonicated to lyse the cells. Cell counts in each sample were calculated based on the assumption that each cell contains 6 pg of DNA[201].

3.2.11 Fastin Assay for Elastic Matrix quantification

A FASTIN assay (Accurate Chemical and Scientific Corp, Westbury, NY) was used to quantify the total elastin deposited by cells as per the manufacturer's protocol. Briefly, 500 μL of the cell lysates harvested in Pi buffer (as discussed in the DNA assay for cell proliferation section) were digested in 1.5 M oxalic acid for 1.5 h at 95 °C to extract soluble alpha-elastin. The digested samples were centrifuged at $14000 \times g$, and the supernatant was transferred to a new 1.5-mL centrifuge tube. The pellet containing insoluble elastin was further digested in 0.25 M oxalic acid (1 h, 100 °C) and centrifuged at $14000 \times g$ to convert it into a soluble form. The sample from the second digestion was pooled with the supernatant from the first digestion. Following the manufacturer protocol, elastin content was calculated using colorimetric absorbance reading at 513 nm. Data were presented by normalizing them with their corresponding DNA contents.

3.2.12 Hydroxyproline Assay for Collagen Quantification

Collagen matrix content was estimated by quantifying total hydroxyproline (OH-Proline) content in the cell culture samples[202,203]. Briefly, for this experiment, 500 μL of the cell lysates harvested in Pi buffer (as discussed in the DNA assay for cell proliferation section) were hydrolyzed in 12 M HCl at 95 °C for 24 h. Cells were then vortexed for 3 min. Colorimetric analysis of OH-proline was done by taking 25 μL of the hydrolyzed sample in a 96-well plate and incubating them with 100 μL of oxidizer solution (mixture of Chloramine T, 1-propanol, citrate buffer) for 30 min in room temperature and then with Erlich's solution (DMAB, 1-propanol, and 70% perchloric acid) for 45 min at 65 °C. All reagents were obtained from Sigma (St. Louis, MO) Absorbance was measured at 550 nm. Collagen amounts were calculated based on the assumption that each fibrillar collagen contains approximately 13.5% w/w of OH-proline.

3.2.13 ELISA for Quantification of Desmosine Crosslinks

Desmosine in the matrix of aHASMC cultures was quantified using a human desmosine ELISA kit (MyBioSource, San Diego, CA). The aHASMCs were harvested in PBS on day 21 and centrifuged at 1000 × g for 15 min and the supernatant was transferred to a new microcentrifuge tube. The cell pellets were subjected to three freeze/thaw cycles and then resuspended in PBS. The resuspended cell pellets were ultrasonicated (20 kHz, 20% amplification, 30 sec on, 10 sec off) and re-pelleted by centrifuging (1000 × g, 15 min, 2-8 °C). A BCA assay was used to quantify the total protein. The samples were then immediately subjected to ELISA assay following the manufacturer's protocol.

3.2.14 MAPK Phosphorylation Antibody Array

To determine the effect of limited SNP dose (100nM vs control) on the expression of phosphorylated (activated) MAPKs, a human MAPK phosphorylation antibody array (ab211061, Abcam) was used. For the experiment, 5×10^4 cells/well were seeded in a 6-well plate and cultured for 14 days. At that time, the cells were serum-starved for 3 h, then treated with a cocktail containing 10 ng/mL of TNF-α and 10 ng/mL of IL-1β, with or without SNP (100 nM) for 10 min, 15 min, and 30 min. Cells that were neither treated with SNP nor with the cytokines served as controls. Cell lysates were harvested in a lysis buffer as provided and recommended by the manufacturer. BCA assay was done to quantify the total protein concentration in each sample. For the MAPK array experiment, briefly, the antibody array membranes were blocked in a blocking buffer (2 mL) for 30 min at 25 °C before incubating them overnight at 4 °C with 150 μg of protein samples. The membranes were washed using the wash buffers and were then sequentially incubated with a detection antibody cocktail and 1× HRP-Anti-Rabbit IgG overnight at 4 °C. Finally, a cocktail of detection antibodies was added to the membrane and the membrane was imaged in ChemiDoc MP (Bio-Rad, Hercules, CA).

3.2.15 Atomic force microscopy (AFM) Analysis for Cellular Forces and Cellura Elastic Response

aHASMCs (10^4 cells per well) were cultured on 2D collagen-coated substrates for up to 48 h in DMEM/F12, containing 0 (Control), 1, 10, or 100 nM SNP. Media was changed once every 24 h with fresh SNP addition. Cells were maintained at 37 °C throughout the live cell nanoindentation assay. An MFP-3D-Bio AFM (Asylum Research, Oxford Instruments, Santa Barbara, CA) mounted on an inverted fluorescence microscope (Nikon Eclipse Ti), and tip-less AFM cantilevers modified by gluing a 5-μm polystyrene bead, were used for the measurements. The spring constant was determined from the force-distance curves using the thermal calibration method in a clean culture dish containing warm media. For each condition, cells were indented between the nuclei and edges, and force curves were obtained at random locations on each cell in force-volume mode at an approach/retraction velocity of 5 μm/s. A Hertz's contact model for spherical indenters, given by $F = 4E_Y\sqrt{R\delta^3}/3(1 - \mu^2)$, was used to determine Young's modulus from these force curves, where F is the indentation force, E_Y is Young's modulus, μ is Poisson's ratio (~ 0.5 for cells), R is the tip radius (2.5 μm), and δ is the indentation depth (~ 500 nm). The force of adhesion (F_{ad}) – the force required to separate the AFM tip and cell surface – was obtained directly from the force-deflection curve during the retraction mode. The tether forces (F_T) were obtained from the force steps displayed in the retraction curves. The apparent membrane tension (T_M), the force needed to deform a membrane, was calculated from such tether forces using $T_M = F_T^2/8\pi^2 k_B$, where k_B is the bending stiffness of membranes (assumed to be ~ 0.1 pN.μm[204]). Similarly, the tether radius (R_T) that describes the plasma membrane to cytoskeleton connection was calculated as $R_T = 2\pi k_B/F_T$. Finally, the mean surface roughness (R_a) of each cell, characterized as the arithmetic mean of the deviations in height from the line mean value, was obtained from randomly selected areas on the cell membrane.

3.2.16 Immunofluorescence (IF)-Based Detection of ECM Homeostasis Proteins

For IF labeling, 15×10^3 cells/well were cultured in a 2-well Permanox chamber slide (Nalge Nunc International, Rochester, NY) as previously published[205]. Briefly, 7 days post-seeding, cells were serum-starved and cytokine-treated, as specified in the experimental plan. The cells were then subjected to SNP treatment for 7 days for signaling MAPK proteins (JNK, p-JNK, ERK, p-ERK) with and without 2-Phenyl-4,4,5,5-tetramethylimidazoline-1-oxyl 3-oxide (PTIO; Sigma) which is a NO scavenger, transmembrane proteins (including MMP2, 9; TIMP1, 2, 4), and 14 days for ECM proteins [elastin (ELN), lysyl oxidase (LOX), fibrillin1 (FBN1)], for total culture times of 14 days or 21 days respectively. At the end of treatment, cells were washed twice with PBS and fixed in 4% w/v paraformaldehyde containing 0.1% v/v Triton X-100 (VWR Scientific, West Chester, PA) for 30 min at room temperature for transmembrane proteins, and with ice-cold methanol for 20 min at 4 °C for ECM proteins. Next, the fixed cells were blocked in 5% v/v goat serum (Gibco) for 30 min. The cells were then incubated overnight with primary antibodies against MMP2, MMP9, TIMP1, TIMP2, TIMP4, ELN, LOX, FBN, JNK, p-JNK, ERK, and p-ERK (Table 3). The expression of these proteins was visualized using either goat anti-rabbit or goat anti-mouse IgG (Alexa Fluor® 594 or Alexa Fluor® 633) (Thermo Fisher Scientific). The nucleus was stained using 4′, 6-diamidino-2-phenylindole (DAPI, Vector Laboratories, Burlingame, CA).

3.2.17 Transmission Electron Microscopy (TEM) to Assess Elastic Matrix Ultrastructure

TEM was used to quantitively assess the newly deposited elastic matrix by aHASMCs and compare them with the untreated controls. aHASMCs were cultured in 2-well Permamox® chamber slides (Sigma) for 21 days. On day 7 of culture, cells were serum-starved and cytokine-injured followed by SNP treatment for 14 days (as described in the experimental plan). On day 21, cells were washed three times with PBS and fixed in a buffer containing 4% w/v paraformaldehyde, 2.5% w/v glutaraldehyde, and 0.1 M sodium cacodylate buffer for 1 h at room temperature, followed by overnight incubation at 4 °C. The samples were then post-fixed with 1% w/v osmium tetroxide for 1 h, dehydrated in 50% - 100% ethanol series, and embedded in the Epon 812 resin before sectioning it and placing them on the copper grids. After that, samples were stained with uranyl acetate and lead citrate before imaging them at multiple magnifications as described in our previously published work[195].

3.2.18 Statistical Analysis

Statistical data analyses were performed using GraphPad Prism®. n=6 cells seeded constructs were used for all experiments (except for cytokine activation, MAPK array, and AFM assessments). statistical comparison between the groups was done using one-way ANOVA or Student's t-test as required. Comparison of different treatment groups with the control was tested with Dunnett's post-hoc analysis and multiple comparisons between the groups were tested with the Tukey-Kramer test. Data are presented as mean ± standard deviation (SD) unless specified, with a *p*-value < 0.05 deemed for statistically significant difference.

3.3 Results

3.3.1 Cell Viability and IC50 of SNP

At SNP doses of 10 mM, 100 µM, 1 µM, 10 nM and 100 pM under low serum conditions (DMEM/F12 with 2% v/v FBS), aHASMC viability were 3.2 ± 0.5 %, 90.8 ± 5.6%, 84.1 ± 8.7%, 83.1 ± 17.4%, and 90.8 ± 5.8%, respectively. Under higher serum conditions (DMEM/F12 with 10 %v/v FBS), cell viabilities at the same SNP doses were 0%, 41.5 ± 6.4%, 55.08 ± 6.4%, 87.3 ± 12.8%, and 96.6 ± 6.7% respectively **(Figure 24)**.

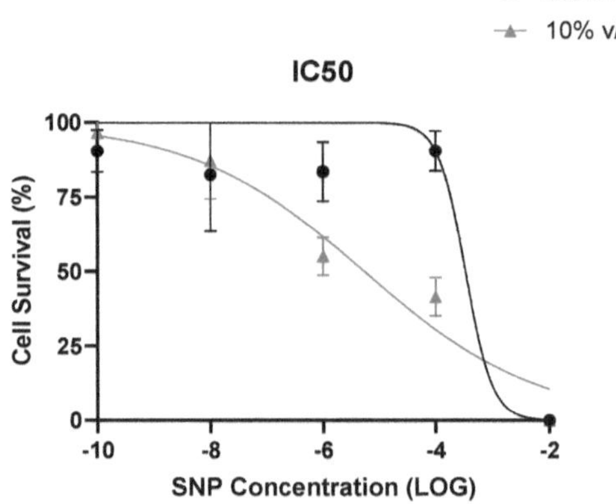

Figure 24: Determination of 50% inhibitory concentration (IC50) of SNP. IC50 of SNP was determined by measuring the concentration-dependent inhibitory effect of SNP on cell survival using non-linear regression (log(inhibitor) vs. normalized response-variable slope) in GraphPad Prism. R-squared values were obtained to be 0.8274 and 0.9226 at 2% v/v FBS and 10% v/v FBS in DMEM/F12 medium

The IC50 values of SNP were calculated to be 0.3 mM and 5.4 µM in low serum and high serum conditions, respectively. Based on this experiment, the acceptable (non-cytotoxic) dose range for *in-vitro* SNP treatment was determined to be between 100 nM and 100pM, as prepared in DMEM/F12 medium containing 10% v/v FBS.

3.3.2   Cytokine Activation of aHASMCs

MMP2 expression increased significantly at 2 h, 3 h, and 24 h of cytokine treatment versus control or those treated with cytokines for only 30 min ($p < 0.0001$) in aHASMC cultures. In addition, MMP2 expression was significantly upregulated in cultures subjected to 2 h, 3 h and 24 h of cytokine exposure (longer exposure) versus 1 h of cytokine exposure ($p = 0.03$). MMP2 expression peaked at 3 h of cytokine exposure and remained unchanged between cultures with longer cytokine exposure times **(Figure 25)**.

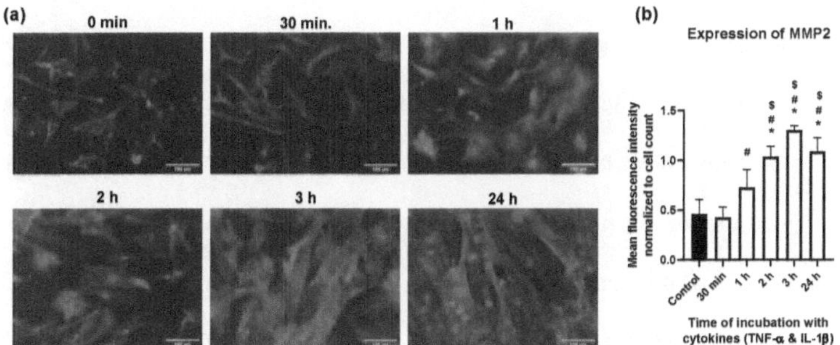

Figure 25: Effect of cytokine exposure duration on the activated phenotype of aHASMCs. (a) IF detection of MMP2 expression (red) in response to cytokine injury on aHASMCs; DAPI-labeled nuclei appear blue. Scale bar = 100 µm. (b) The fluorescence intensity of MMP2 expression from the IF images was quantified, normalized to the respective nuclei count, and represented as mean ± SD. *, # and $ denote p = 0.05 compared to controls, 30 min of cytokine treatment, and 24 h of cytokine treatment respectively (n = 4 cultures/case)

3.3.3 Effect of SNP on ECM Homeostasis and aHASMC Phenotypic Marker Proteins

Figure 26 shows the gene expression in cytokine-injured aHASMC cultures following treatment with a range of SNP doses. **Figure 26a** shows the expression of SMC marker genes. Smooth muscle alpha-actin (*ACTA)* and desmin (*DES)* expression by aHASMCs was downregulated at all SNP doses ($p = 0.001$ and 0.02 vs control, respectively), and myosin heavy chain (*MYH11)* expression was reduced at all SNP doses except 100 pM ($p = 0.05$ vs control). The gene expressions of end-stage contractile SMC phenotypic markers, smoothelin (*SMTH*), and calponin (*CNN*) remained unaffected by SNP.

Furthermore, *MMP2* gene expression was significantly decreased upon SNP treatment versus controls ($p < 0.05$ vs control: **Figure 26b**). Among TIMPs **(Figure 26b)**, *TIMP1* gene expressions remained unchanged at all dosages, while *TIMP2* was significantly upregulated only at 100 nM ($p = 0.006$) and *TIMP4* was downregulated at 100 pM ($p = 0.03$ vs control) but remained unchanged at higher doses. Elastin (*ELN*) gene expression was significantly higher at the 100 nM SNP ($p = 0.05$ vs. control) and lysyl oxidase (*LOX*) gene expression was upregulated at 100 pM and 100 nM ($p = 0.03$ vs control) **(Figure 26b)**. In addition, the gene expression ratio of *TIMP1* to *MMP2* was upregulated at 10 nM (p=0.01), and 100 nM (p=0.001) by ~1.8 ± 0.4 and ~2.03 ± 0.2-fold respectively, and the gene expression ration of *TIMP2* to *MMP2* was upregulated at 100 nM (p=0.0001) by ~5 ± 0.8-fold. However, there was no significant change in *TIMP4* to *MMP2* gene expression ratios with SNP treatment. On the other hand, the gene expression ratio of *ELN* to *COL3A1* was significantly upregulated at 100 nM by ~5 ± 0.5-fold (p=0.03) whereas, gene expression of *ELN* to *COL1A1* did not change significantly.

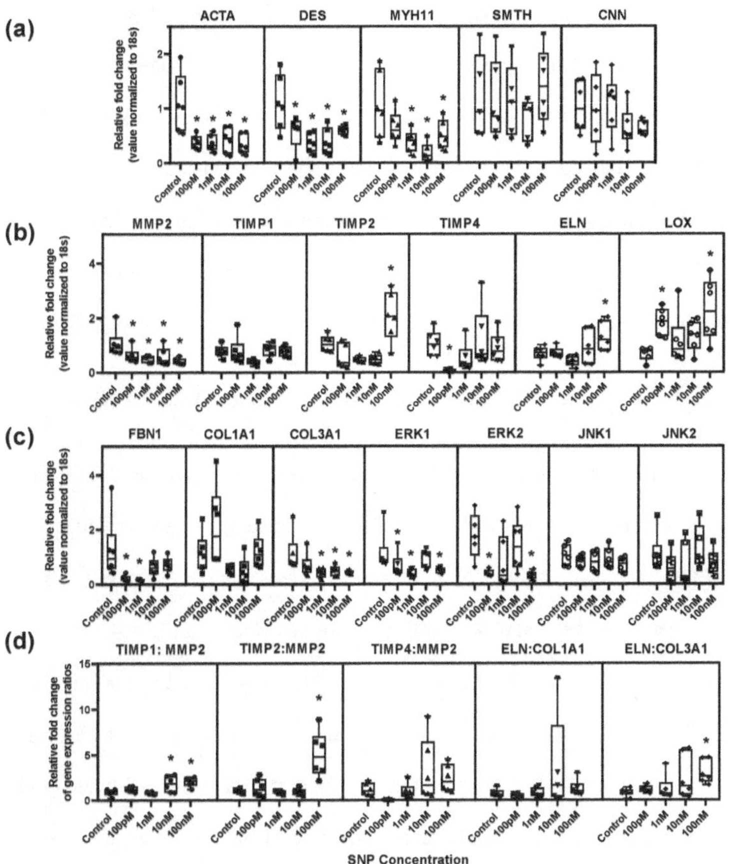

Figure 26: Panels (a-c) SNP effects on gene expressions of various phenotypic markers, ECM homeostasis proteins, and MAPK proteins in aHASMC cultures. Panel d shows the gene expression ratio of TIMP1 to MMP2, TIMP2 to MMP2, TIMP4 to MMP2, ELN to COL1A1 and ELN to COL3A. Data were presented as mean ± SD (n = 6 cultures/condition). * Denotes p < 0.05 compared to untreated controls for each gene

100

In addition, relative gene expression of fibrillin (*FBN1*) was downregulated at 100 pM and 1 nM of SNP (p = 0.006 vs. control) but remained unchanged at higher doses, and collagen type I alpha 1 (*COL1A1*) genes were unaffected by SNP treatment **(Figure 26c)**. In contrast, collagen type III alpha 1 (*COL3A1*) was significantly downregulated at all SNP doses (p = 0.03 vs. control) except at 100 pM SNP **(Figure 26c)**. Among various MAPKs **(Figure 26c),** gene expression of *ERK1* was downregulated at all SNP doses (p = 0.01 vs control) except at 10 nM. *ERK2* gene expression was downregulated at 100 pM and 100 nM (p = 0.02 vs control), whereas *JNK1* and *JNK2* gene expression remained unchanged at all SNP doses.

3.3.4   Effect of SNP on Expression of ECM Homeostasis Proteins

The dose-dependent effects of exogenous SNP on the synthesis of key ECM homeostasis proteins (MMPs, TIMPs), cell signaling MAPK proteins (JNK, ERK), and ECM proteins (LOX, FBN1) **(Figure 27)** were semi-quantitatively assessed using WB analysis. At all tested doses, SNP suppressed MMP2 levels (p = 0.001 vs control) **(Figure 27a)**. Although TIMP1 (28 kDa) and TIMP2 (24 kDa) remained undetected in WBs, TIMP4 was detected in two distinct bands – 26 kDa and 62 kDa **(Figure 27b)**. The expression of TIMP4 (both isoforms) appeared higher in SNP-treated cultures, but this increase was not statistically higher than in control cultures. At the analysis time points, the expression of MAPK proteins including JNK **(Figure 27c)**, ERK1 (44 kDa), and ERK2 (42 kDa) **(Figure 27d)** was not significantly altered by SNP treatment. Similarly, FBN1 (312 kDa) was not significantly different **(Figure 27e)**; however, LOX (47 kDa) was upregulated at 100 pM SNP dose (p = 0.006), 1 nM dose (p = 0.04) and 100 nM dose (p =

0.004) (**Figure 27f**). Additionally, gelatin zymography of MMP2 showed significant

downregulation at 1 nM, 10 nM, and 100 nM (p=0.04) SNP dose.

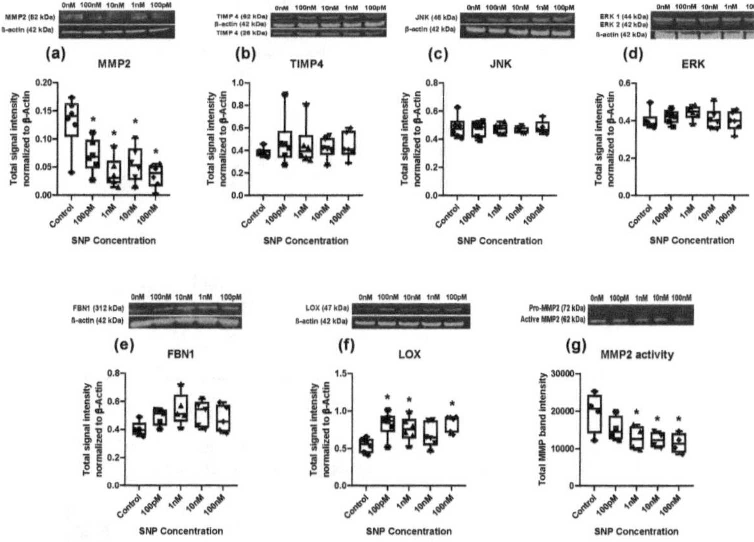

Figure 27: Dose-dependent effects of SNP on ECM homeostasis proteins as
determined by WB analysis. (a-f) The total signal intensity of each analyzed protein was
further normalized to β-actin expression and shown, along with representative WB gel
blots. (g) Representative gelatin zymography showing total MMP2 activity. Y-axis
represents total MMP2 band intensity obtained from the gels (n=4). Data were presented
as mean ± SD of results obtained for n = 6 cultures/condition with statistical differences
(p < 0.05) versus untreated controls indicated by *

3.3.5 Effect of SNP on aHASMC Gene Expression Profile at Pro-Regenerative/Anti-Proteolytic Dose

RT-PCR and WB results indicated significant matrix regenerative and anti-proteolytic

benefits of SNP in aHASMC cultures at the 100 nM dose. A human qPCR gene analysis array was performed at this singular dose to assess SNP effects more broadly on expression profiles of different functionally grouped genes.

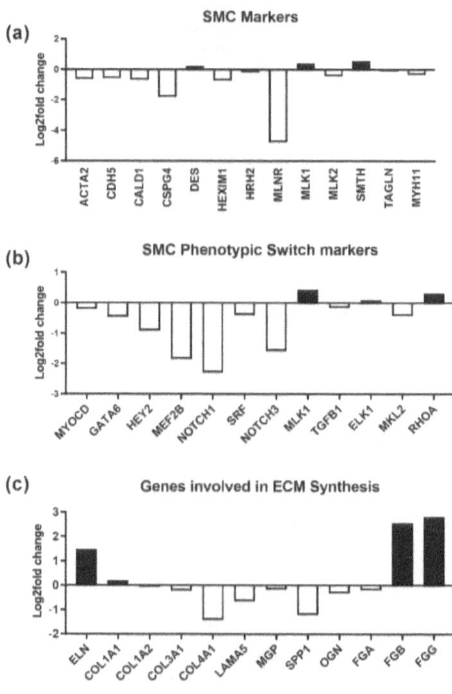

Figure 28:   A human SMC biology qPCR array was used to determine the effects of various doses of SNP on the gene expression profiles of functionally-grouped SMC markers. The fold-changes in the relative gene expression of various SMC markers (a), SMC phenotypic switch markers (b), and ECM synthesis markers (c) were analyzed by the ΔΔCt method. Bar graphs above the baseline value (represented by the line at y=0) represents upregulation and below the baseline represents downregulation

Among the analyzed genes, the contractile SMC markers *ACTA* and Caldesmon 1 (*CAD1*) were downregulated upon SNP treatment (**Figure 28a**). SNP also downregulated genes known to induce synthetic-like SMC phenotype and regulate the growth,

103

proliferation, and migration of SMCs, such as myocardin (*MYOD*), GATA binding protein 6 (*GATA6*), Hairy/enhancer-of-split related with YRPW motif protein 2 (*HEY2*), monocyte enhancer binding factor 2B (*MEF2B*), Notch receptor 1 (*NOTCH1*), and Notch receptor 3 (*NOTCH3*) (**Figure 28b**). Furthermore, there was an increase in *ELN* expression and comparatively lower expression of collagen type I (*COL1A1* and *COL1A2*) and collagen type III (*COL3A1*) genes (**Figure 28c**). Collagen type IV gene (*COL4A1*) expression was highly reduced.

3.3.6 Effect of SNP on Cell Viability

We determined the cytotoxicity of SNP doses in a range of 100 nM to 1 μM to select a safe dose range for our dose escalation study done to determine the effects of SNP on cell proliferation and elastic matrix synthesis. Results from the LIVE/DEAD™ assay showed a significant reduction in cell viability at 1 μM dose of SNP ($p = 0.0001$). Cell viability was

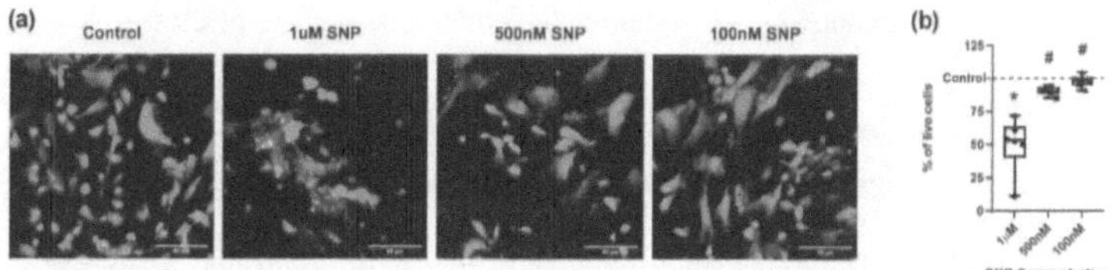

Figure 29: LIVE/DEAD analysis of cytotoxicity of SNP on aHASMCs in an escalated dose range of 100 nM to 1 μM. (a) Fluorescence images of cultured aHASMCs stained with calcein-AM (live, green) and ethidium homodimer-1 (dead, red). Scale bar: 50 μm. (b) A boxplot showing the percentage of the live cells in each case (treatment vs control). Data were normalized to untreated controls (100% live cells as shown by the dotted line). * Denotes statistical significance ($p < 0.05$) compared to controls, # denotes significance ($p < 0.05$) compared to 1 μM SNP

not adversely impacted at 500 nM and 100 nM of SNP relative to controls but was significantly higher than in the cultures treated with 1 μM of SNP ($p = 0.0001$ vs 1 μM)

104

(**Figure 29**). The percentage of live cells in cultures treated with 1 µM, 500 nM, and 100 nM of SNP was 50.1 ± 20.6%, 90.3 ± 3.2%, and 98.1 ± 4.6% respectively.

3.3.7   Effect of SNP on Cell Proliferation and ECM Synthesis

Based on the initial findings of LIVE/DEAD™ assay and the pro-regenerative and anti-proteolytic effects of SNP at the 100 nM dose, SNP effects on matrix synthesis were evaluated at this and higher doses (250 nM, 500 nM). No significant difference was seen in cell proliferation between control and 100 nM SNP treated cultures although higher SNP doses induced significantly robust proliferation of aHASMCs versus controls ($p = 0.002$ and 0.005 for 250 nM & 500 nM, respectively) and 100 nM SNP dose ($p = 0.01$ and 0.02 for 250 nM & 500 nM, respectively) (**Figure 30a**). The total elastic matrix content in the SNP treated cultures were all significantly higher than in the controls ($p = 0.0004$, 0.0001, 0.0001 vs. controls for 100, 250, and 500 nM of SNP respectively (**Figure 30b**)). There were no significant SNP-dose-dependent differences in total elastin amounts within the groups. On a cell count-normalized basis, elastic matrix amounts were deemed significantly higher than controls only in cultures treated with 100 nM of SNP ($p = 0.01$ vs control) (**Figure 30c**). On the other hand, the hydroxyproline assay did not detect any collagen in the samples. In addition, the total desmosine (normalized to total protein concentration) obtained from the ELISA showed significant upregulation at 100 nM and 500 nM of SNP ($p = 0.03$ and $p = 0.04$ vs control) in our Dunnett's post hoc analysis (**Figure 30d**).

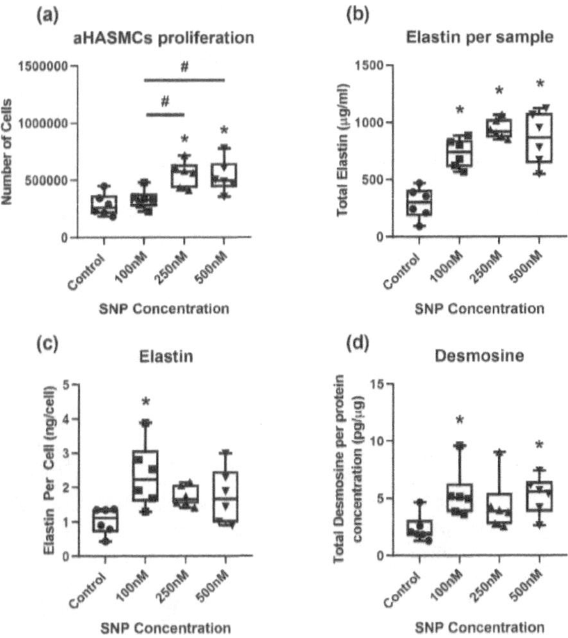

Figure 30: The effects of SNP dose escalation, beyond the basal efficacious dose (100 nM), on aHASMC proliferation, elastic matrix synthesis, and cross-linking was shown. The effect of various SNP doses on cell proliferation (a), total elastic matrix synthesis (b), elastin amounts normalized per cell (c), and desmosine crosslinker amounts normalized to total protein (d) were quantified from various assays and represented as mean ± SD (n = 6 cultures/condition). The differences deemed statistically significant (p < 0.05) compared to controls and 100 nM dose were indicated by * and #, respectively

3.3.8 Effect of SNP on MAPK Proteins

The human MAPK phosphorylation antibody array experiment results are indicated in the heat map shown in **Figure 31a**. The heat map indicates increased expression of MAPK signaling proteins when treated solely with cytokines (TNFα and IL-1β). In all cases, the peak expression of these MAPKs occurred at 15 min and 30 min of cytokine exposure. Such upregulation was inhibited by the administration of 100 nM of SNP together with cytokine exposure, as shown by the decreased expression of these MAPKs (**Figure 31b**). The expressions of JNK, ERK, AKT, MEK, MKK3, MKK6, and mTor were all inhibited by 100 nM of SNP at all tested exposure times. In addition, GSK-3 (GSK3α and GSK3β), RSK1/2, and the transcription factor, CREB expression also decreased with SNP treatment.

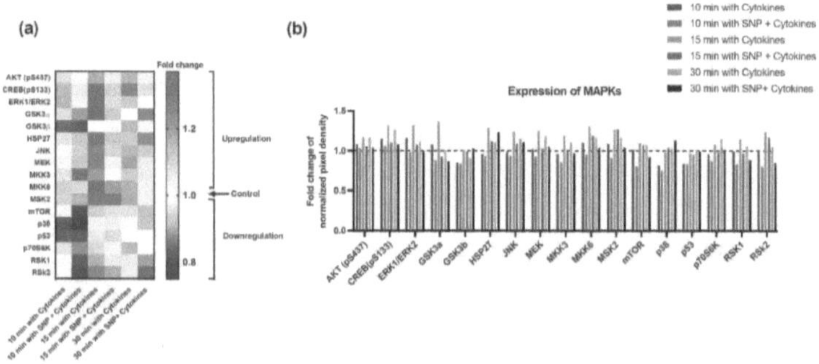

Figure 31: Expression of phosphorylated MAPKs as a function of time in cytokine-injured aHASMC cultures with or without SNP treatment. (a) A heat map of the results from a human MAPK phosphorylation array experiment. The red color represents higher MAPK expression (upregulation), blue represents lower MAPK expression (downregulation), while white (indicated at 1 in the heat map) is the normalized expression of MAPKs in control cultures. Cultures received cytokine alone or cytokines and SNP for various durations, while control cultures received none. (b) Representative bar graph of the human MAPK phosphorylation experiment (n = 2 repeats per condition). The mean pixel density of each target protein was normalized to the pixel density of the positive control. The y-axis in the graph represents the fold change obtained by normalizing the normalized pixel density to that in controls. The dotted line marked along y=1 represents the fold change of the untread aHASMC controls (no cytokines, no SNP). Legend: CREB = cAMP response element-binding protein, ERK= Extracellular signal-regulated kinase, GSK3= Glycogen-synthase kinase 3, HSP27= heat shock protein 27, JNK= c-Jun N-terminal Kinase, MEK/MKK= Mitogen-activated protein kinase kinase, MSK= Mitogen and stress-activated kinase, mTOR= Mechanistic target of rapamycin, RSK= Ribosomal S6 kinase

3.3.9   Effect of SNP and NO Scavenger on MAPK Proteins

To further verify the role of SNP in regulating MAPKs (most specifically JNK, ERK, p-JNK, and p-ERK as these are abundantly expressed in AAAs) and to demonstrate that NO is the key regulator of this phenomenon, we performed IF-based labeling of these proteins in our cytokine injured aHASMC cultures with and without SNP treatment (100 nM) and NO scavenger (**Figure 32**) for 15 min. Our IF results were consistent with our MAPK array results indicating cytokine treatment (10 ng/mL of TNF-α and 10 ng/mL of IL-1β) caused a significant upregulation in ERK and p-JNK ($p<0.01$) compared to control aHASMCs (without cytokine exposure) (**Figure 32b**). Although expression levels of JNK and p-ERK were not significant with cytokine exposure, an increasing trend in the expression levels was still observed when exposed to cytokines. The parallel exposure of these cytokine-injured aHASMCs with 100nM of SNP for 15 min significantly inhibited the expression of ERK ($p=0.002$), p-ERK ($p=0.02$), JNK ($p=0.001$), and p-JNK ($p=0.04$). Conversely, the addition of 200 nM PTIO, a NO scavenger, overturned the inhibitory effect of SNP significantly on JNK ($p=0.006$), p=JNK($p=0.03$), and restored their expression levels to control values or in between control and cytokine-treated values. Also, the trend in the increase or decrease of these MAPKs with cytokine treatment and with the introduction of SNP and PTIO was similar in all proteins despite their significant differences or no-significant changes among the groups. In addition, the increase or decrease in the MMP2 expression in our IF experiment (**Figure 32(a-b)** can be correlated to the expression of these MAPKs which suggests that the inhibitory effect of MMP2 was likely via the inhibition of MAPKs and was governed by released NO.

108

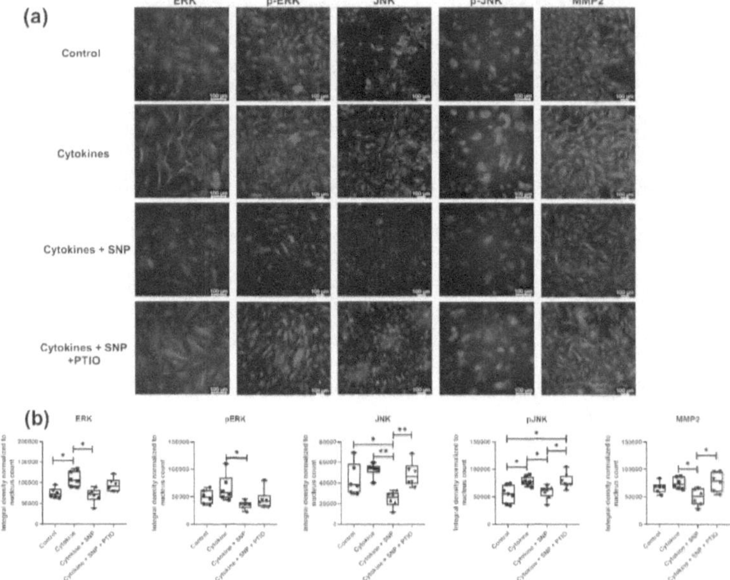

Figure 32: Immunofluorescence-based demonstration of the involvement of NO in inhibiting non-phosphorylated and phosphorylated MAPKs. Panel a) shows the IF-based labeling of ERK, p-ERK, JNK, p-JNK, and MMP2 in cytokine-injured, cytokine and SNP-treated, and cytokine, SNP and PTIO (NO scavenger) treated aHASMCs. Panel b) shows the representative integral density boxplots of the respective IF images. Scale bar = 100 μm. Data are presented as mean ± SD of values obtained from n = 6 cultures/condition * Denotes (p < 0.05), ** denotes (p<0.005)

3.3.10 Effect of SNP on Biomechanical Characteristics of aHASMCs

Single cell nanoindentation measurements were obtained to quantify the biophysical and biomechanical characteristics of live human aHASMCs under different SNP dosing conditions. The SNP dosages selected were based on cell survival and IC50 studies discussed earlier. The modulus of elasticity (E_Y) decreased significantly at 10 nM and 100 nM exposure compared to control or 1 nM SNP dose (**Figure 33a**; $p < 0.05$ for 10 nM vs.

100 nM). The average E_Y in control cultures was 20.9 ± 7.7 kPa and exposure to 100 nM SNP reduced it by ~ 60% to 9.64 ± 4.1 kPa.

Similarly, the forces of adhesion were not significant at 1 nM SNP vs. control but were significantly reduced at 10 nM and 100 nM SNP (**Figure 33b**; $p < 0.05$ for 10 nM vs. 100 nM and vs. control). The baseline adhesive forces in control cultures were 1.87 ± 0.13 nN. The tether forces (F_T) on the cell surface were significantly reduced with the addition of SNP ($p < 0.05$ vs. controls), even at as low as 1 nM concentration (**Figure 33c**). The baseline tether forces for control cultures were 218.8 ± 14.3 pN, while that in the presence of 100 nM SNP dropped to 75.8 ± 12.6 pN (~65% drop vs. controls).

The membrane tension and tether radius were calculated from the tether forces and trends were along expected lines as in F_T. With increasing SNP concentration, membrane tension decreased significantly (**Figure 33d**) while the tether radius proportionately increased (**Figure 33e**), compared to controls. The baseline membrane tension in control cultures was 6.07 ± 0.8 nN/μm while the tether radius was 2.91 ± 0.19 nm. Cell roughness measurements showed that the cell surface of aHASMCs turned significantly rougher with the addition of 100 nM SNP, while lower SNP dosages had no significant effect compared to controls (**Figure 33f**). For all the measured parameters, no significant changes were noted at longer culture durations (24 h or 48 h) in control aHASMC cultures without SNP.

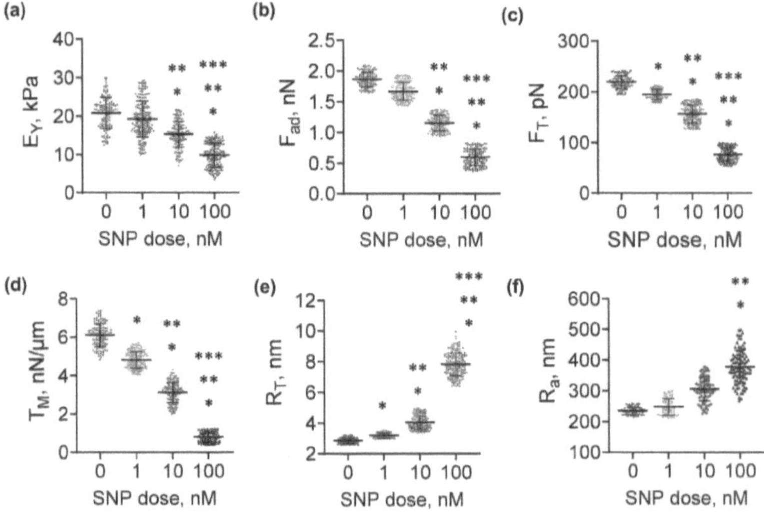

Figure 33: Dose-dependent effect of higher SNP doses (1 nM, 10 nM, 100 nM) on cellular elastic response as determined by AFM. (a) Elastic modulus of the cells (E_Y) calculated by applying Hertz model to force–indentation curves ($128 \leq n \leq 205$ cells/ condition). (b) Adhesion forces measured from the force–indentation curves during retraction mode ($109 \leq n \leq 167$ cells/ condition). (c) Tether forces measured from the force–indentation curves during retraction mode ($119 \leq n \leq 188$ cells/ condition). (d) Membrane tension on the cell surface (T_M) calculated from the tether forces using $T_M = F_T^2/8\pi^2 k_B$. (e) The radius of tether (R_T) calculated from F_T values using $R_T = 2\pi k_B/F_T$. (f) The surface roughness parameter (R_a) on the cell surface is measured using AFM tip ($77 \leq n \leq 98$ cells/ condition) for control and SNP-exposed cells. Data presented as mean ± SD, with statistical significance deemed for $p < 0.05$ and indicated by * for differences vs. control, ** for differences vs. 1 nM dose of SNP, and *** for differences vs. 10 nM dose of SNP

3.3.11 Effect of SNP on the Expression of ECM Homeostasis Proteins as Seen in IF

Representative IF staining of aHASMCs for expression of MMP2, TIMP1, TIMP2, TIMP4 and ELN, LOX, FBN1 were shown in **Figure 34**. MMP2 expressions in cultures treated with SNP (100 nM) were significantly suppressed relative to control cultures ($p = 0.03$) and were seen as a diffused band surrounding the nuclei. SNP did not necessarily affect TIMP1 expression. However, TIMP2 and TIMP4 were found to be significantly higher in SNP-treated aHASMCs ($p = 0.001$) and were seen to be expressed in a diffused manner around the cell nuclei, similar to MMP2. ELN and LOX expression was also significantly higher in SNP-treated cultures versus controls ($p = 0.004$). There were no apparent differences in FBN1 expression between control- and SNP-treated cultures.

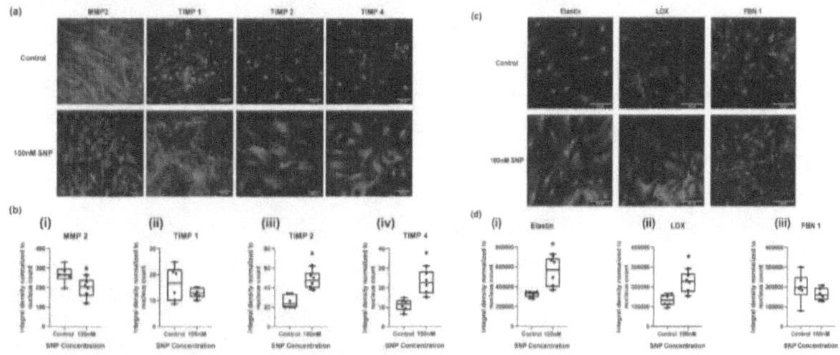

Figure 34: Immunofluorescence detection of ECM homeostasis proteins in SNP-treated and untreated aHASMC cultures. Panels a and b indicate representative IF images of MMP2 and TIMPs (TIMP1, TIMP2, TIMP4), and boxplots showing mean fluorescence intensities for the respective proteins obtained by analysis of these images. Panels c and d show confocal images of elastin, LOX, and FBN1 expression and boxplots indicating quantification of fluorescence intensities. Scale bar = 100 μm. Data are presented as mean ± SD of values obtained from n = 6 cultures/condition, * denotes statistical significance compared to the untreated control and deemed for p < 0.05

3.3.12 SNP Effects on Elastic Matrix Ultrastructure

TEM images showed evidence of a dense elastic matrix composed of newly formed, mature elastic fibers (black arrows) in the ECM in the 100 nM SNP-treated group (**Figure 35a**). In contrast, control aHASMC cultures exhibited very few, nascent, and often fragmented elastic fibers (red arrow; **Figure 35b**).

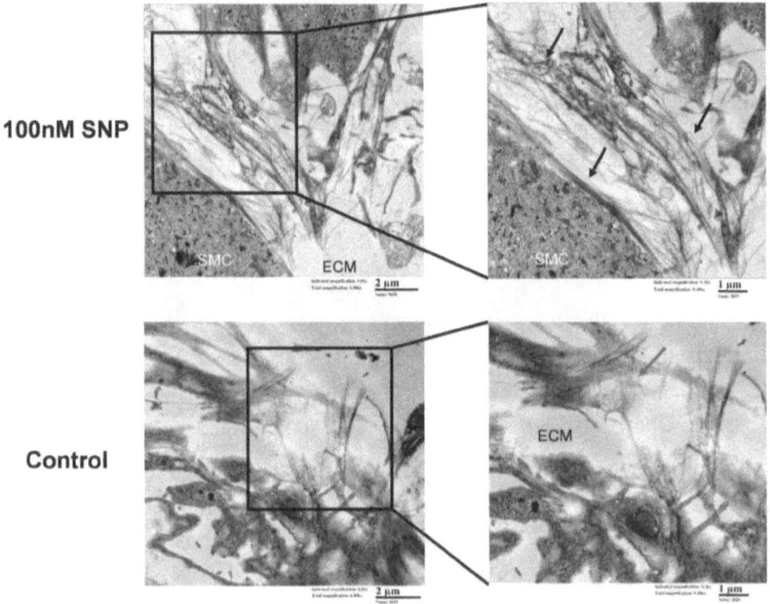

Figure 35: The effect of SNP treatment on elastic matrix ultrastructure formed in cell cultures was imaged using transmission electron microscopy. (a) Ultrastructure of thick, newly formed, elastic fibers composed of elastin coacervates (tropoelastin) shown in black arrow in 100 nM SNP-treated aHASMC cultures after 14 days of exposure. (b) Thin and fragmented elastic in untreated control group (red arrow)

3.4   Discussion

AAAs represent localized expansions of the abdominal aorta due to naturally irreversible degradation and loss of wall elastic matrix caused by chronically activated MMPs following initial injury stimuli. AAA pathophysiology is exacerbated by intrinsic abnormalities in elastic fiber neoassembly and repair, chronic inflammatory response, the switch of medial SMCs to a diseased phenotype, and the association of NO signaling dysfunction[11]. In this study, we sought to assess if delivery of SNP (NO donor drug) is a useful treatment modality to augment elastic matrix regenerative repair and anti-proteolytic effects and to promote SMC phenotypes capable of directing elastic matrix regeneration. We investigated these aspects in a cytokine injury model of human aneurysmal SMCs or aHASMCs. Pro-inflammatory cytokines, such as TNF-α and IL-1β which regulates various inflammatory signaling in the cells, are known to be upregulated in AAA milieu[62]. In our study, the cytokine injury model (exposure of aHASMCs to a cocktail of 10 ng/mL of TNF-α and 10 ng/mL of IL-1β) was adopted to a) mimic inflammatory diseased state even after their isolation from physiological conditions and b) to determine how effective SNP treatment would be in terms of elastic matrix regenerative repair under these disease-mimicking conditions. Our results indicate that 3 h of cytokine exposure has a maximal effect on aHASMCs' MMP2 production, which is the key to ECM degradation.

Next, to establish a safe, working SNP dose range, the IC50 (the half maximal inhibitory concentration of SNP on cell survival) in aHASMC cultures was measured in 2% v/v FBS (low serum) and 10% v/v FBS (higher serum) containing medium. The far lower IC50 value observed in the high serum (5.4 μM) compared to low serum conditions (0.3 mM) (**Figure 24**) is likely due to the increased generation of reactive oxygen species (ROS) under higher serum conditions, which consequently causes more DNA damage and cell death[206,207]. On the other hand, SNP, at higher concentrations activates MAPKs, such as p38, through cGMP independent pathway which further triggers pro-inflammatory activation of the MMPs [208]. That said, in our working SNP dose range identified based on the IC50 value at high serum conditions, overall cytotoxic effects were rather limited (<15% cell death; **Figure 24**). Although SNP, which is an FDA-approved hypertensive drug commonly known as Nitropress™, can activate stress-induced MAPK pathways and be associated with cyanide and ROS toxicity, our data suggest that in the working dose range in the high serum condition, SNP likely has the anti-MAPK effect and low cyanide-related cytotoxicity. The reduced-cytotoxicity effect of SNP was further verified by our LIVE/DEAD™ assay results which showed that cell death was not enhanced even at an escalated dose range of 1 µM and 100 – 500 nM (**Figure 29**). However, toxicity profiles of SNP at various serum levels should be thoroughly assessed to shed more light on SNP-induced *in-vitro* cytotoxicity. Since low serum condition is not physiologically relevant, to reflect *in-vivo* conditions more closely, we adopted higher serum conditions for *in-vitro* assessment.

Next, we investigated the effects of SNP on the expression of ECM homeostasis proteins in our cultures. Several *in-vitro* studies have suggested a possible connection between NO deficiency and chronic overexpression of the elastolytic MMPs (MMP2 and 9), the most abundant endopeptidases in the AAA wall, which critically drive elastic matrix degradation [209,210]. To date, a spate of published studies has also demonstrated that inhibiting MMP2 and MMP9 can attenuate inflammatory tissue damage following injury[211], and limit chronic MMP-mediated ECM breakdown and loss[212]. Consistent with earlier findings, our results showed SNP delivery to significantly downregulate MMP2 expression (**Figure 26b**, **Figure 27a**, **Figure 32**, and **Figure 34 (a,b)**) and MMP2 activity (**Figure 27g**). MMP2 expression in treated aHASMCs (**Figure 25a**, **Figure 27a**, and **Figure 34**), as seen in our IF images, shows diffused and spread patterns, which is in coherence with another published study[141]. The lack of any discernable effects on MMP9 expression (data not shown), despite the evidence of NO-mediated MMP9 inhibition in HUVEC and rat mesangial cells [213,214], is likely due to a very low intrinsic expression of

MMP9 (protein and gene) in cell culture which is likely because of the absence of macrophages and macrophage-generated reactive nitrogen oxide species (RNOS) linked to triggering MMP9 activation[213]. As a next step, we propose to investigate possible SNP effects on MMP9 in a more complex *in-vitro* culture model incorporating matrix debridement with macrophages which we have published[215].

Our results further indicate that the inhibition of MMP2 can be linked to the significant increase in TIMP2 and TIMP4 (inhibitors of MMPs) (**Figure 26b** and **Figure 34(a-b)**). However, no significant change was seen in TIMP4 western blots, but, it colocalized with active MMP2 bands **(Figure 27b)** suggesting the potential inhibitory effect of TIMP4 against MMP-mediated proteolysis likely by fine-tuning active- MMP activities as suggested by few studies[216,217]. Despite the substantial increase in TIMP2 gene and protein expression with both RT-PCR and IF at 100nM of SNP, we were unable to detect TIMP2 with WB while TIMP1 expression did not change in RT-PCR **(Figure 2b)** and in IF **(Figure 34(a-b))** and remained undetected in WB like TIMP2. This outcome is likely due to the inherent difference in the probe sensitivity and binding efficiency of TIMP1 and TIMP2 to their respective antibodies, and low protein yield from our cultures which limited protein loading onto our WB gels. In terms of gene expression ratio, there was a significant increase in TIMP1 to MMP2 and TIMP2 to MMP2 ratio showing the potential anti-MMP effect of SNP (at 100 nM) in our aHASMC cultures **(Figure 26d)**.

The anti-MMP effect of SNP we observed could involve activation of either cGMP-dependent pathways, cGMP-independent pathways, or both by the NO released from SNP[218,219]. While the primary focus of this study lies in assessing SNP effects in promoting elastin homeostasis in the context of AAAs, we have sought to broadly understand the underlying mechanisms, specifically the involvement of the cGMP-independent pathway. This pathway regulates various cellular transcription factors and consequently modulates gene and protein expressions of the cells via S-nitrosylation of cysteine residues of the receptors of the MAPK pathways [220]. Among several MAPKs, the JNK and ERK signaling pathways have been most implicated in AAAs[16,195]. Our findings suggest significant downregulation in *ERK1* and *ERK2* gene expression (**Figure 26c**) but no difference in gene and protein expression of other *MAPKs*, e.g., *JNK1*, and *JNK2* with SNP treatment. This is probably due to the transient expression of these MAPK proteins and their relatively shorter half-life, which renders their detection in long-term treated (7 days) cultures challenging[221]. Therefore, to further demonstrate the role of SNP in regulating transiently expressed MAPKs, we performed a MAPK array experiment at short cytokine and SNP exposure times (< 30 min) in our culture model. This MAPK array provides the screening of a broader spectrum of MAPKs which likely have a direct or indirect association with the inflammatory milieu of proteolytic disorders such as in AAAs.

Most of the MAPKs such as AKT, CREB, ERK1, ERK2, JNK, MEK, MKK3, MKK6, MSK2, mTor, p38, p53, RSK1, and RSK2, are implicated in proteolytic disorders, with JNK and ERK being the primary MAPKs that drives the formation and progression of AAAs[16,222,223]. While our WB result showed no significant differences in JNK and ERK expression at a 7-day time point, downregulation of these MAPKs was observed in the MAPK array experiments at time points of 0-30 min (**Figure 31**). To further verify the role of cytokine and SNP exposure in downregulating MAPKs (specifically JNK, p-JNK, ERK, and p-ERK) and to determine if these effects were mediated by NO released from SNP, we performed IF-based labeling of these MAPKs which showed significant upregulation and downregulation of MAPKs with cytokine exposure and with parallel SNP treatment respectively **(Figure 32(a-b))**. However, this effect was completely overturned with the addition of NO scavenger, PTIO, which suggests that the SNP-mediated MAPK inhibition was regulated by NO. In addition, the expression of MMP2 was correlated with MAPK expressions which suggests that the anti-MMP effect in our aHASMC cultures is regulated via MAPK attenuation. Moreover, SNP treatment caused the downregulation of other MAPKs as seen in our MAPK array results. GSK-3 is considered to be at the crossroads of various other signaling pathways including EGFR, Ras, AKT, and mTor, and is known to control Nf-$\kappa\beta$ activity via IkappaB kinase (IKK)/ Nf-$\kappa\beta$ essential modifier (NEMO)regulation [224,225]. Similarly, CREB is a transcription factor that regulates various gene expressions in response to the cAMP changes and has also been shown to regulate expressions of MMP2 in other cell types[226]. Other isoforms of MAPKs such as MEK, MKK3, MKK6, MSK2, p38, p53, RSK1, and RSK2 also control a wide range of biological functions and therefore increase the range of action regulated by the active forms of MAPKs mentioned above to drive the inflammatory response[227]. Overall, our MAPK array experiment has demonstrated that SNP has inhibitory effects on various MAPKs which perhaps occurs through disorganization of actin filaments possibly via cGMP-dependent signaling and/or by attenuation of NOTCH signaling pathway [228,229]. NOTCH signaling pathways have been previously shown to specifically activate the MEK, ERK, and AKT pathways[230,231]. On this basis, we hypothesize that the SNP-mediated MAPK inhibition in our study is mediated by disruption of the actin cytoskeleton (**Figure 26a** and **Figure 27a)** and *NOTCH* deactivation **(Figure 28b)**. Also, NOTCH signaling is associated with the phenotypic modulation of VSMCs[12,232,233]. Increased activity of NOTCH1 and NOTCH3 have been shown to promote SMCs proliferation, and collagen synthesis, and induce a synthetic SMC phenotype through downstream regulation of CHF1/HEY2 [63]. Downregulation of *HEY2, NOTCH1*, and *NOTCH3* in our qPCR array **(Figure 28b)** and our experimental findings on cell proliferation particularly at 100 nM SNP **(Figure 30a)** suggest that the cells are not assuming a highly synthetic SMC phenotype that could potentially promote hyperplasia in a AAA wall milieu. This is also supported by our RT-PCR results showing unchanged expression of end-stage SMC contractile phenotypic markers (*SMTH* and *CNN* **(Figure 26a)**) between SNP-treated and untreated groups. The decrease in *COL3A1* gene expression **(Figure 26c)** in RT-PCR and lower expressions of collagens (COL) in the qPCR array **(Figure 26c),** whose expression is elevated in SMCs of a synthetic SMC phenotype[234], also supports the inference that SNP exposure does not trigger a highly synthetic SMC phenotype. On the other hand, as anticipated, there was a significant downregulation in *ACTA, DES*, and *MYH11* **(Figure 26a)** genes encoding contractile apparatus proteins as NO donor compounds have been frequently shown to downregulate contractile apparatus genes and induce muscle relaxation by downregulating interactions of the actin-tropomyosin-myosin complex involved in the sliding filament mechanism of cell contraction[235,236]. Collectively, our gene expression analysis and biochemical assay results indicate that at 100nM, SNP did not induce synthetic phenotypes in culture but did promote a more relaxed cell state.

To investigate the phenotypic changes in aHASMCs in response to NO exposure, we performed AFM analysis. We had two hypotheses: a) will NO exposure soften the cells, and if so, in a dose-dependent manner, and b) does NO exposure cause any change to the cell surface (glycocalyx)? Live cell indentation of aHASMCs with AFM **(Figure 33)** showed a significant reduction of Young's modulus and cell surface adhesive forces at SNP doses of 10 nM and 100 nM suggesting aHASMCs acquired softer characteristics with SNP treatment. Similarly, tether force which is dependent on membrane adhesion as well as cytoskeleton adhesion was significantly reduced with increasing SNP dosage in our study suggesting decreased cytoskeletal density in the aHASMC cultures[237]. The decreased gene expression of *ACTA, MYH11,* and *DES* in our gene study further verifies that the decrease in these forces is likely because of a decrease in the cytoskeletal protein expression with SNP treatment[238]. Furthermore, the radius of tether and surface roughness increased with increasing SNP concentrations, possibly via a similar mechanism explained above and via modulation of cell surface proteins[239]. Overall, our study showed that the forces required to separate the non-functionalized polystyrene bead-modified AFM tip from the cell surface were strongly dependent on the SNP concentration in the culture media. aHASMCs turned softer from a stiffness standpoint, while their surfaces turned pliable and rough in the presence of SNP similar to what was noted in prior study[239]. The no significant change in the control cultures at longer time points verifies that the differences seen in these parameters were mediated by SNP. In addition, the glycocalyx might also be undergoing some changes in response to NO exposure, as shown by the decreased adhesion force, although such changes are tedious to quantify using other techniques.

In healthy vessels, the turnover of structural ECM proteins (e.g., elastin and collagen) is very low due to low MMP activity and an intrinsic balance between MMPs and TIMPs. Differently, the chronic upregulation of MMPs in the AAA wall leads to increased fragmentation of both elastic fibers and collagen fibers to cause ultimate wall weakening and rupture[240]. Elastic matrix regeneration is particularly challenging due to the poor intrinsic elastin synthesis capacity of adult and diseased VSMCs and their impaired ability to assemble mature elastic fibers. Different from elastin, vascular SMCs robustly synthesize collagen thereby increasing the collagen-to-elastin ratio either by collagen synthesis and/or disproportionate degradation of non-collagenous structural proteins[241]. Our findings demonstrate that elastic matrix synthesis by aHASMCs is significantly enhanced with SNP treatment as suggested by increased *ELN* gene expression at 100 nM SNP **(Figure 26b),** protein expression **(Figure 34(c-d))** and increases in total matrix elastin amounts and on a per cell basis **(Figure 30 (b-c)** at 100 nM. Elastin may sometimes appear to be localized within or around the cell, likely due to the fact that most of the extracellular matrix proteins are produced by SMCs in the cell or on the cell surface in their precursor form (elastin and collagen) where they begin to form crosslinks and are eventually deposited on the extracellular matrix[242,243]. To elucidate further on this, we performed TEM of our cultured aHASMCs to visualize the ultrastructure of the deposited fibers and verify if the newly formed elastic matrix is deposited in the ECM or within the cells. TEM images in **Figure 35** show that SNP treatment stimulated elastic fiber formation and the majority of which was deposited in the ECM space with some fibers being around the cell membrane.

While collagen protein amounts were below the threshold for reliable detection, the significant increases seen in the *ELN/COL3A1* ratio **(Figure 26d)** at the pro-elastogenic/anti-proteolytic SNP dose (100 nM) suggests progress towards restoring ECM homeostasis with SNP treatment as collagen accumulation is primarily associated with an adverse fibrotic response of vascular SMCs and contribute to the vascular stiffness[244]. A possible reason for having no detected collagen in our cultures could be due to the highly diseased nature of aHASMCs (harvested from severe AAA tissues). At later stages of AAA progression when an aneurysm reaches a rupture-prone stage, chronic proteolytic degradation of both collagen and elastin occurs and the cells gradually lose their ability to restore these elastic matrix assembly proteins[245]. Moreover, a published study has shown that SNP treatment in vascular SMC inhibits collagen production by 42%[246] which might also explain the reason for below threshold collagen levels in our aHASMC cultures treated with SNP. Furthermore, the coacervation and crosslinking of elastin precursors by LOX provide structural integrity to the ECM by forming strong intermolecular covalent bonds between elastin precursors[247]. LOX (precursor, 50kDa) produced by SMCs are hydrolyzed into their active form that promotes cross-linking of fibrous ECM proteins such as elastin and collagen into a non-soluble state[248]. The inactivation of the *LOX* gene resulted in the formation of large aortic aneurysms, cardiovascular dysfunction, and perinatal death in LOX knockout (LOX $^{-/-}$) mice[249]. Conversely, an increase in LOX has been shown to improve elastic matrix crosslinking[195,205]. Consistent with these outcomes, our observed increases in the *LOX* gene **(Figure 26b)** and LOX protein expression **(Figure 27f and Figure 34(c-d))** with SNP treatment correlated positively with increased expression of desmosine **(Figure 30d).** Desmosine is a crosslinker molecule essential for elastic matrix formation, crosslinking, and maturation. The formation of desmosine occurs within the formation of precursor tropoelastin. During development, SMCs produce tropoelastin on the cell surface where LOX helps in the oxidative deamination of lysine residues of tropoelastin to form allysine that further reacts with other lysine residues of tropoelastins to form desmosine [242,250]. Our observed increases in desmosine content with SNP treatment of cultures can be inferred to be indicative of increased cross-linking of the elastin. And, once the crosslinking process of many soluble elastin precursors is done, the elastic matrix is finally deposited on the ECM for further maturation and crosslinking[251].

Elastic fiber assembly is a complex, multi-step process orchestrated by several key proteins and glycoproteins. Fibulins (FBLNs), particularly Fibulin 4 and 5, facilitate crosslinking of tropoelastin to form coacervates that engage with a pre-scaffold of FBN1 glycoprotein to promote elastic fiber assembly[252]. However, despite SNP-induced increases in elastin and LOX, in the tested dose range, SNP did not impact gene and protein expression of FBLNs (data not shown) and FBN1 **(Figure 26c, Figure 27e, and Figure 34(c-d))**. In addition, the aHASMCs used in our study were harvested from severe AAA tissues, as previously described, and they have an intrinsically poor ability to regenerate both elastin and collagen. Moreover, we had difficulties growing these cells in glass chamber slides as they started to detach immediately after 7 days of culture in some culture dishes. Despite these challenges, the TEM experiment (aHASMCs cultured for 21 days) shows evidence of elastic matrix formation in aHASMC cultures treated with 100 nM SNP **(Figure 35)**. The newly formed elastin can be seen as fibers (as shown by the black arrow (top images)) in the ECM and around the cell (red arrow) which is consistent with the ultrastructure shown by Robb et al[253]. On the other hand, the control cultures had very few traces of elastin regeneration, and those which were there were thin and sporadic (white arrow). Since our TEM micrographs indicate increased elastic fiber formation in SNP (100 nM)-treated *in-vitro* cultures relative to control **Figure 35)**, this outcome is likely driven primarily by increases in tropoelastin synthesis, and desmosine and LOX-mediated crosslinking rather than by increases in our assessed elastic fiber assembly proteins such

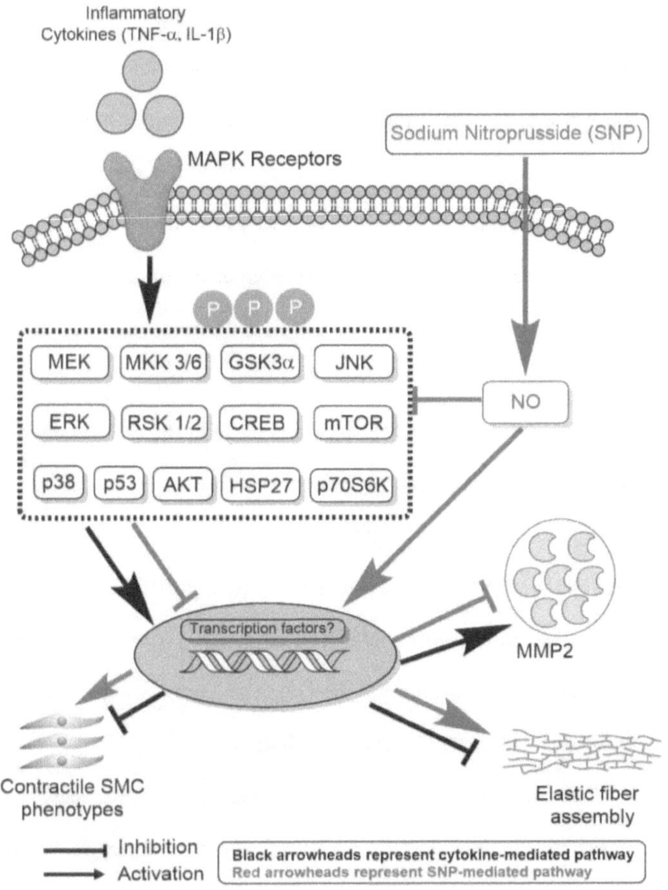

Figure 36: Hypothesized MAPK-mediated mechanistic pathway engaged by SNP for anti-proteolytic and pro-elastogenic regulation of ECM homeostasis in aHASMCs. Arrows indicate activation and T lines represent inhibition. Question mark indicates that the critical transcription factors remain to be identified. Inflammatory cytokines (TNF-α and IL1β) activated MAPK signaling. SNP attenuated these MAPKs to or below the control value which in turn attenuated MMP2 (gene and protein expression), increased elastic matrix components (elastin, LOX, desmosine) and promoted contractile SMC phenotypes

as fibrillin and fibulins. In addition to the improvement in the elastic matrix assembly in aHASMCs with SNP treatment, various studies have reported that SNP increases compliance of the aortic wall consequently decreasing the arterial stiffness and providing mechanical stability to the aortic stretch and recoil function[254,255]. As collagen is the major determinant of matrix stiffness, the decreased expression of collagen genes, no detection of collagen in our biochemical assays, upregulation of elastin to collagen gene expression ratio, and upregulation of elastic matrix deposition and crosslinking suggest that SNP treatment does not probably contribute to ECM stiffness, rather, it might improve the elastic function of the ECM. Since microcalcification of the arterial wall is related to arterial stiffness[256], and SNP suppresses calcification by decreasing calcium current in the cells[257], it is expected that SNP likely reduces calcification of the vessel wall. However, to determine how SNP contributes to the long-term stabilization of the mechanical properties of the ECM, more extensive studies in *in-vitro* (3D) cultures and *in-vivo* studies might be required. In a nutshell, the anti-proteolytic and pro-elastogenic effects of SNP as seen in our *in-vitro* study are summarized in **Figure 36**.

The work reported in this chapter showed that SNP treatment is useful to restore ECM homeostasis and modulate the phenotype of human aneurysmal SMCs *in-vitro* cultures. SNP upregulated elastic matrix assembly, crosslinking, and maturation and concurrently inhibited MMPs via NO-mediated MAPK inhibition. In addition to this, we have also demonstrated the ability of SNP to promote contractile sub-populations of SMCs in culture conditions which promote elastic matrix synthesis. However, one potential drawback of exogenous SNP delivery is that NO is immediately released in the aqueous microenvironment and being a short-lived molecule, quickly oxidizes into less effective nitrite and nitrate in aqueous conditions. Thus, in the next chapter we have separately designed SNP delivering nanoplatforms for controlled delivery of SNP, which will also offer opportunities for localized drug delivery at efficacious doses within the AAA wall *in vivo*. The proposed approach has the potential to delay the growth of small AAAs to a rupture stage that mandates risky surgery for mostly older AAA patients.

CHAPTER IV: Novel Lipid Nanoparticle-Charged Grafts (LCGs) for Localized Sodium Nitroprusside Delivery Enhancing In-Vitro and Ex-Vivo Regenerative Repair of Abdominal Aortic Aneurysms (AAAs)

4.1   Introduction

As previously discussed, AAA is a severe vascular disorder characterized by chronic proteolytic degradation of the vascular wall and often is associated with macrophage infiltration and cytokine production, activation of SMCs for MMP secretion, degradation of elastin and collagen resulting in disrupted, disorganized and tortuous fibers, and depletion of SMCs and ECs[258]. Dysfunctional NO signaling plays a critical role in AAA pathophysiolgy[11,60]. Elastic matrix degradation and loss is by and large viewed as naturally irreversible[53,245,259]. In our earlier aim, we demonstrated that the exogenous administration of the NO donor drug, SNP, stimulates *in-vitro* aHASMC cultures to facilitate elastic matrix regeneration[260]. Additionally, it confers anti-proteolytic benefits by inhibiting MMP2 expression and upregulating TIMPs expression, while also inducing SMCs to exhibit contractile phenotypes in culture[167,168,260].

As discussed previously, the standard approach to AAA management involves passive monitoring of AAA growth or surgical intervention at a more rupture imminent stage. Small AAAs are monitored using imaging-based surveillance and managed with oral drug-based treatments to slow down elastin degradation. In contrast, large AAAs typically require surgical intervention. These surgical approaches are often linked to mortality rates as high as 10 percent[261], and they pose greater risks to patients with symptomatic aneurysms[262]. The periadventitial graft placement, designed for multifaceted purposes including providing mechanical support and facilitating drug delivery with drug-encapsulated nanocarriers, has the potential to substantially reduce the morbidity and mortality rates associated with these high-risk interventions. This is of particular significance given the elevated prevalence of AAAs in elderly patients over 65 years of age, who often present with coexisting comorbidities[9,263].

As discussed earlier, oral drug-based therapies have shown limited promise in slowing, stopping, or reversing AAA pathophysiology likely due to the uncertain pharmacokinetics of the drugs in the gut[25,178]. To address these challenges, we have developed an innovative solution with lipid nanoparticle-charged grafts (LCGs) which combines drug-delivery liposomes or lipid nanoparticles (LNPs) with a vascular graft made from PCL that can be peri-adventitially placed around the aneurysmal aorta segment. While LNPs offer superior drug delivering capabilities due to their biocompatibility, biodegradability, size tunability, and capacity to encapsulate a wide range of drug molecules and/or siRNAs for gene knockdown as shown in our prior work[264], slow degrading polycaprolactone (PCL), a synthetic polymer, has been shown to significantly enhance vascularization and efficient regeneration of the functional tunica media, making it an ideal candidate as an vascular graft substitute[265,266]. PCL also exhibits impressive non-immunogenic properties and has been shown to provide mechanical properties that are adequate for use as small diameter vascular grafts when applied in rat and mouse abdominal models[267,268]. Furthermore, leveraging well documented robust affinity between biotin and neutravidin, we developed LCGs that incorporate biotinylated LNPs (bLNPs) onto biotinylated PCL (bPCL) meshes via neutravidin bridging. This design enables the SNP-loaded bLNPs to achieve localized and sustained SNP release when they are incorporated onto the bPCL graft. The versatility of LCGs offers a wide range of drug delivery options.

This chapter details the a) formulation and characterization of LNPs, b) biotinylation of LNPs using 1,2-Distearoyl-sn-glycero-3-phosphoethanolamine (DSPE) PEG-Biotin, c) creation of LCGs, d) encapsulation of SNP, and e) characterization of encapsulation efficiency, long-term SNP release kinetics, and the *in-vitro* and *ex-vivo* advantages of LCGs, highlighting their potential as an alternative treatment for AAAs in the future.

4.2   Materials and Methods

4.2.1   Formulation and Biotinylation of Lipid Nanoparticles (LNPs)

To initiate the process, cationic lipid nanoparticles (LNPs) were produced through the thin-film hydration method as previously detailed in our published work[264]. In this method, a mixture composed of 1,2-dioleoyl-3-(trimethylammonium) propane (DOTAP), dioleoylphosphatidylethanolamine (DOPE), and cholesterol, at a molar ratio of 0.5/0.5/0.5 (DOTAP/DOPE/Cholesterol), was created in a round bottom flask. For biotinylation of LNPs, 40 mol % DSPE PEG-Biotin (Avanti Polar Lipids, Alabaster, AL) was added to this mixture of DOTAP/DOPE/Cholesterol. Subsequently, the mixture was subjected to a rotary evaporator (R-215, Buchi Corporation, New Castle, DE) placed in a water bath at 50 °C for 10 minutes, with rotation at 280 RPM and 300 mbar pressure. This process led to the formation of a thin film. To eliminate any residual chloroform, the resulting film was vacuum dehydrated in a desiccator overnight. Hydration of the film was achieved by adding water, followed by vortexing for 1 h at room temperature and allowing overnight swelling at 4 °C. The LNPs were then extruded 20 times through a 100nm polycarbonate Avanti Mini-Extruder (Avanti Polar Lipids, Alabaster, AL) to ensure a uniform size distribution ranging between 100 and 200 nm.

4.2.2 Characterization of LNPs

Size (100-200 nm), charge (<50 mV), and polydispersity index (PDI, ideally <0.5) was measured using dynamic light scattering (DLS) in a Zetasizer nano ZS (Malvern Panalytical, United Kingdom)[269]. For size and PDI assessment, LNPs with and without biotin were diluted at a 1:1000 v/v ratio in RNase-free water, while for charge measurement, the LNP suspension was diluted at a 1:100 v/v ratio. Measurements were conducted with predefined parameters, enabling the Zetasizer to execute automated runs for all evaluations (at least 10 runs per parameter). Size, charge, and PDI characterization were carried out across a minimum of three batches, each with three replicate runs. The degree of biotinylation on bLNPs was quantified using the QuantTag Biotin quantification kit (Vector Labs, Newark, CA) coupled with a subsequent washing procedure to remove any unbound PEG-Biotin. This washing process involved centrifugation through a 100 kDa centrifuge filter at 12,000 rpm for 15 minutes, repeated three times, and maintained at 4 °C.

4.2.3 SNP Encapsulation within bLNPs and Evaluation of Encapsulation Efficiency

To encapsulate SNP, a thin film of the lipid mixture, including DSPE PEG-Biotin as described earlier, was hydrated (2 h) with SNP prepared in RNase-free water at a concentration of 29.795 mg/mL, resulting in a final 100 mM stock concentration. The resultant mixture of SNP and thin lipid film, referred to as SNP-bLNP mixture, underwent 20 consecutive extrusion cycles in a mini extruder equipped with a 100 nm polycarbonate filter, as outlined earlier. Following the extrusion process, the LNPs encapsulating the SNP were filtered using a 100 kDa centrifuge filter. This filtration step was carried out at 5000 rpm and 4 °C for a duration of 15 min in 3 repeat cycles. Encapsulation efficiency was quantified by analyzing the flow-through and measuring the concentration of this flow-through using Greiss Reagent. This was followed by subtraction of the concentration of the flow-through from the initial stock concentration also determined using Greiss reagent. The calculation of encapsulation efficiency was conducted across three separate batches, with each batch having a minimum of triplicate readings to ensure robustness and accuracy of the results.

4.2.4   SNP Release Study

The *in-vitro* release of SNP from bLNPs was evaluated in PBS at 37 °C, over a 45-day time period. In brief, 5 mg of SNP-bLNPs was dissolved in 1 mL of PBS within a microcentrifuge tube and placed in an incubator under continuous shaking to avoid sedimentation of bLNPs at the bottom. Release kinetics were determined at specific time points over a period of 45 days. At each designated time point, bLNPs were centrifuged at 12000 rpm for 15 minutes at 4 °C. A 60 µl aliquot was frozen (-20 °C) at each specified time point until colorimetric detection of SNP. An equivalent of 60 µl of PBS was added to compensate for the loss in total volume after aliquoting. The relative SNP release kinetics was determined by measuring nitrite levels (in percentage) using the Greiss reagent kit (Promega, Madison, WI), following manufacturer instructions.

4.2.5 Mathematical Curve Fitting of SNP Release Data

The SNP release profiles obtained from release study provide valuable insights into SNP release mechanisms and inform us about the required drug loading for targeted 100 nM release at a specific time, aligning with our previously established optimal dosage for elastic matrix regeneration[260]. To assess the fit of our experimental results, we employed the Korsmeyer-Peppas (KP) model, a semi-empirical model capable of accurately forecasting the theoretical drug release at specific concentrations and time intervals[270]. This model helped determine the required SNP loading onto bLNPs to achieve a 100 nM SNP release for our cell-based experiments.

$$C_T = C_\alpha k t^n \qquad \text{equation 1}$$

In this equation, C_t represents the amount of SNP released at 't', C_α represents the total amount of SNP released by that time, k is the drug release rate constant, which accounts for the geometrical and structural aspects of the drug release system, and 'n' represents the release exponent. If n<0.43, then the drug release follows classical Fickian diffusion, if n>0.85, then the releases is governed by Type II transport involving lipid swelling and/or erosion-based drug release. And if 0.43>n<0.85, then the drug release is based on non-Fickian transport[271].

4.2.6 Culturing Cryopreserved aHASMCs

aHASMCs were harvested and frozen from tissue biopsies obtained during open surgical repair procedures at the Cleveland Clinic, in accordance with methods detailed in our previously published research[260,272]. The aHASMCs were subsequently passaged and cultured in a medium comprised of Dulbecco's modified Eagle's medium and Ham's F-12 medium (DMEM/F12; Thermo Fisher Scientific, Waltham, MA), supplemented with 10% fetal bovine serum (FBS; Gibco, Waltham, MA) and 1% penicillin-streptomycin (Pen-Strep; Thermo Fisher Scientific). The cells were maintained in a humidified incubator at 37 °C with 5% CO2. Experiments were conducted using cells from passages 3 to 8.

4.2.7   Conjugation of bLNPs on a Biotinylated PCL Graft Using Neutravidin Bridge

Biotinylated PCL (bPCL) grafts were fabricated by our collaborators, the Chow Lab at Lehigh University, and developed as described in their published work[273]. To summarize, bPCL was synthesized through a two-step procedure. Initially, biotin was modified with Boc-protected ethylenediamine using a carbodiimide amide-forming reaction. Subsequently, the Boc group was removed from the biotin-ethylenediamine, followed by a second carbodiimide amide-forming reaction with PCL (80 kDa). Finally biotinylated PCL (bPCL) formed by this technique was used for conjugating bLNPs to make lipid NP charged graft (LCG).

Prior to conjugation, bPCL grafts were rinsed 10 times in PBS. DyLight 488-labeled neutravidin (ThermoFisher, Waltham, MA) was then introduced at a concentration of 0.1 mg/mL onto the bPCL grafts placed within a 24-well plate. Incubation of the bPCL grafts occurred for 1 h at room temperature with gentle shaking. After incubation, the bPCL grafts underwent five washes in Tris-buffer saline with Tween20 (TBS-T). Next, the bPCL grafts were blocked using a 3% BSA solution in TBS-T buffer for 30 min. Following blocking, the grafts were incubated with DiR-labeled bLNPs at a concentration of 0.2 mg/mL, with a neutravidin-to-bLNP ratio of 1:2. This incubation continued for 1 h. The grafts were washed five times before being imaged on a Leica DMi8 microscope (Leica, Wetzlar, Germany) in the far red and green fluorescence channels. PCL graft and LNPs lacking biotin were employed as controls.

4.2.8   Assessment of bLNP Cytotoxicity

aHASMCs were cultured under standard conditions using DMEM/F12 supplemented with 10% v/v FBS and 1% v/v Pen-Strep until confluency. Afterwards, cells (15×10^3 cells/well) were grown in 12-well plates. On the 7th day, cells underwent a 3 h serum starvation, followed by exposure to inflammatory cytokines (3 h), TNF-α (10 ng/mL) and IL-1β (10 ng/mL), which are often associated with inflammatory milieu of AAAs[62]. Subsequently, the cells were exposed to bLNPs at concentrations of 0.1 mg/mL, 0.25 mg/mL, 0.5 mg/mL, and 1 mg/mL for 24 h. The cells were then rinsed with PBS and assessed using a Live/Dead assay (Invitrogen, Waltham, MA) following the manufacturer's instructions.

4.2.9   Cytotoxicity Assessment of LCGs

Cytotoxicity of LCGs was assessed in both contact and non-contact modes in an aHASMC culture model. To evaluate cytotoxicity in the cell, contact model, 24-well plates were coated with silicon elastomer, allowing cells to attach exclusively on LCGs while preventing their attachment elsewhere in the well. A two-component silicone elastomer (Sylgard 184) was mixed in a 10:1 ratio of silicon elastomer to crosslinker. This mixture, sufficient to cover half of each well, was applied and cured in a fume hood at room temperature for 24 h. After ensuring the elastomer's substantial curing, 5 mm × 5 mm bPCL punches were placed on top of the curing silicon elastomer, ensuring that the bPCL remained on the surface rather than sinking into the elastomer. The silicon elastomer with bPCL was allowed to cure for an additional 24 h. Following this, the silicone-coated well plates with bPCL placed on top underwent three repeats 1 h water wash cycles. Subsequently, the plates were sterilized with 70% ethanol (2 h) and exposed to UV radiation for 30 minutes within a biosafety cabinet for maximum sterilization. In the next step, bLNPs were conjugated to the bPCL graft as described above except that the bPCL (or PCL) graft, in this experiment, were incubated with 3 w/v % BSA for 3 h instead of just 30 min. Then, LCGs conjugated with bLNP at 0.1 mg/mL, 0.25 mg/mL, and 0.5 mg/mL were formulated and 15×10^3 cells/well were seeded directly onto the LCG graft. The cells were allowed to attach for 72 h before performing LIVE/DEAD assay for cytotoxicity.

In the non-cell contact model, 15×10^3 cells per well were initially seeded in a 24-well plate and allowed to proliferate for 24 h. Following this incubation, the cells were exposed to LCGs conjugated with bLNP at concentrations of 0.1 mg/mL, 0.25 mg/mL, and 0.5 mg/mL. To prevent direct contact between the LCGs and the cells, the LCGs were positioned on cell inserts having a semipermeable bottom. After 72 h, cytotoxicity was evaluated using a LIVE/Dead assay.

4.2.10 RT-PCR Analysis to Assess Anti-proteolytic and Pro-elastogenic Effects of LCGs

Real-time polymerase chain reaction (RT-PCR) was performed to determine the gene expression of key genes associated with elastic matrix homeostasis and aberrations thereof in the AAA wall, including *MMP2*, *TIMP 1*, *TIMP2*, *TIMP4*, *COLIIIA1*, *ELN*, and *LOX*. Briefly, 30×10^3 aHASMCs/well were cultured in a 6 well plate and allowed to attach for 7 days. On day 7, aHASMCs were serum starved (3 h) and cytokines treated (3 h) with the cocktail of 10 ng/mL of each of TNF-α and IL-1β. Immediately, we treated aHASMCs with 15×15 mm SNP LCGs (i.e SNP encapsulated bLNPs (0.25 mg/mL) conjugated onto bPCL) and with blank LCGs (i.e. blank bLNPs conjugated onto bPCL) in a non-contact model using cell inserts for 7 days, simulating their placement periadventitially in an in vivo setting for future applications, thus excluding a contact model in our experiments. We compared our results with the control cultures that were untreated with LCGs. On day 14, the aHASMCs were harvested, and total mRNA was extracted following the manufacturer's guidelines using the RNeasy Mini Kit (Qiagen, Valencia, CA). mRNA quantification was performed with a Nanodrop 2000 (Thermo Fisher Scientific, Wilmington, DE). Subsequently, 200 ng of total mRNA was reverse-transcribed using the iScript cDNA Synthesis Kit (Bio-Rad, Hercules, CA), and RT-PCR was carried out with the SYBR Green master mix for cDNA amplification. Relative gene expression was determined using the ΔΔCt method, as described by Livak et al[198]. The cycle threshold (Ct) values of the target genes were double normalized to the average Ct values of their respective 18S and GAPDH genes and then normalized again to the no-treatment control to calculate gene expression fold change.

4.2.11 Western Blot for Protein Analysis of Key ECM Homeostasis Proteins

The analysis of relative protein expression for the genes mentioned in the RT-PCR section was performed via Western Blotting. Briefly, aHASMCs 50×10^3 aHASMCs/well were cultured in a 6 well plate and allowed to attach for 7 days followed by serum starvation and cytokine treatment as detailed earlier. The application of SNP LCGs (0.25 mg/mL of bLNPs) and blank LCGs to aHASMCs were carried out using a non-contact method with a cell insert. On the 14th day (7 days post-treatment), aHASMCs were harvested in RIPA buffer (Thermo Fisher Scientific), supplemented with 1% vol/vol Halt protease inhibitor and phosphatase inhibitor (Thermo Fisher Scientific). Total protein quantification was performed using the Bicinchoninic acid (BCA) assay, and 4 µg of protein was loaded into NuPAGE Bis-Tris gels for electrophoresis. Subsequently, the gels were transferred to a nitrocellulose membrane, followed by blocking and incubation with primary antibodies for MMP2, TIMP1, TIMP2, TIMP4, LOX at a 1:1000 vol/vol dilution, and secondary antibody (IRDye® 680LT goat-anti-rabbit) at a 1:15,000 vol/vol dilution, as previously described in our recently published work[260]. Membrane imaging was conducted using an Odyssey® XF imager (LI-COR, Lincoln, NE).

4.2.12 Decellularization and Elastase-Induced ECM Disruption in Porcine Carotid Arteries

To create an *ex-vivo* model AAA model, porcine carotid arteries (PCAs) were first subjected to decellularization, following established protocols[274]. Briefly, the PCAs were initially subjected to a 10-minute DI water wash on a shaker which was repeated three times to get rid of the residual blood. A 5 mm section was taken and frozen in OCT compound (-80 °C) to be used as native controls. Subsequently, remaining PCAs, each approximately 3 cm in length, were placed in a 15 mL tube and immersed in a 0.5 v/v % Triton X-100 solution, undergoing a 24 h incubation at room temperature on a shaker. The

PCAs were then washed for 2 h and immersed in a 0.25 v/v % SDS solution on a shaker for 24, 36, 48, and 72 h in a longitudinal experiment to determine the extent of decellularization and the effect of detergents on the elastic matrix. After each decellularization period, the decellularized PCAs (dPCAs) underwent a 48 h washing step to remove residual detergents. Subsequently, they were preserved in OCT compound, and frozen. The PCAs that were not frozen in the OCT compounds were stored in -20 °C for future use.

To create a AAA *ex-vivo* model which more closely evokes the elastic matrix - disrupted ECM milieu in the AAA vessel segment in vivo, dPCAs that underwent 24 h of decellularization with Triton X-100 followed by a 36 h decellularization with SDS (which was used for further experiments) were incubated with 96 units of porcine pancreatic elastase ($\geq$4.0 units/mg protein; Millipore Sigma, Burlington, MA) at 37 °C for short periods (1 h, 2 h, and 3 h), considering their relatively small size. Both test groups (elastase-treated) and control groups (decellularized for 24 h in Triton X + 36 h in SDS) were embedded in OCT and the generated 15-μm thick sectionssubject to histolgical analysis.

4.2.13 Cryo-sectioning and Histological Analysis for Cell Nuclei/Elastin Quantification

Cryo-sectioning of the OCT frozen tissue was done in Bright OTF5000 cryostat. In summary, native and dPCAs were cryosectioned to a thickness of 15 μm and affixed to glass slides for subsequent histological analysis. The slides were stained following or previous study[275]. All PCA sections were fixed with ice-cold acetone for 7-10 min and allowed to air dry at room temperature. Subsequently, the PCA sections underwent two 5-

minute washes with PBS. They were then immersed in a 0.05% w/v solution of Pontamine Sky Blue (MP Biomedicals, Irvine, CA) for 30 minutes, followed by three rinses with water. The prepared slides were laid flat, and a drop of Vectashield, which contained the nuclear stain 4',6-diamidino-2-phenylindole (DAPI) (Fisher Scientific, Hampton, NH), was applied over the PCA sections. A coverslip was placed on top, and visualization was carried out using a Keyence BZ-X Microscope (Keyence, Osaka, Japan). The effectiveness of cell removal and the retention of elastic matrix were assessed by counting the remaining cells (identified by blue DAPI staining) and measuring the elastin content based on the fluorescence intensity of Pontamine sky blue at the chosen time points in the native and dPCA.

4.2.14 Cytotoxicity of Decellularized PCAs

Cytotoxicity assessment of the dPCAs was conducted utilizing a LIVE/DEAD assay kit. Initially, a 12-well plate was coated with a two-part silicon elastomer, as previously described. A 30 µm section of dPCA decellularized for 36 h followed by 2 h of elastase incubation was positioned onto the PDMS and secured to prevent tissue flotation. Before cell seeding, the PCA-containing PDMS-coated plates were subjected to a 1 h wash with DI water. Subsequently, the tissues were sterilized with ethanol for 30 minutes and then exposed to UV light for 15 minutes. Prior to aHASMC seeding, the dPCAs were incubated overnight at 4 °C in DMEM F-12 (with 10% v/v FBS and 1% v/v Pen-strep). Following this incubation, 15×10^3 aHASMCs were directly seeded onto the dPCA, and an additional 200 µL of DMEM F-12 media was added. The aHASMCs were allowed to adhere and proliferate for 72 h, and cytotoxicity was assessed using the LIVE/DEAD assay, as previously described.

4.2.15 Immunofluorescence (IF) Visualization of Select ECM Homeostasis Proteins

The expression of key elastin homeostasis proteins was further assessed using IF. Briefly, 15×10^3 cells/well were cultured in a 12-well plate. On the 7th day, aHASMCs underwent serum starvation for 3 h and were then exposed to a cytokine mixture consisting of 10 ng/mL of TNFα and 10 ng/mL of IL-1β, prepared in DMEM F-12 for 3 h. The cells were subsequently treated with LCGs conjugated with 0.25 mg/mL of bLNPs for 7 days.

For the IF analysis on the re-cellularized PCA (rPCA), a 12-well plate was first coated with a two-part silicon elastomer, as described earlier. A 30 μm section of dPCA, which had undergone 36 h of decellularization followed by 2 h of elastase incubation, was carefully placed onto the PDMS and securely fixed to prevent tissue flotation. The plate was then left to be cured completely overnight in a fume hood at room temperature. Subsequently, the plates were sterilized as detailed in the previous section. Next, 15×10^3 cells were directly seeded onto the PCA and allowed to adhere for 72 h. To mimic the non-contact drug delivery model, LCGs containing 0.25 mg/mL of bLNPs were introduced using insect pins onto the graft and treated for 7 days.

After the end of the treatment period, well plates were washed twice with PBS and the cells were fixed for MMP2 in 4% w/v paraformaldehyde containing 0.1% v/v Triton X-100 for 30 minutes at room temperature, while for elastin cells were fixed with ice-cold methanol for 10 minutes at 4 °C. Following fixation, the cells were blocked for 1 h and then incubated overnight with primary antibodies against MMP2 and ELN. The expression of these proteins was visualized using secondary antibodies (goat anti-rabbit or goat anti-mouse IgG - Alexa Fluor 594 (Thermo Fisher Scientific). Nuclei were stained with 4',6-diamidino-2-phenylindole (DAPI; Vector Laboratories, Burlingame, CA) and observed under a microscope for imaging.

4.2.16 Statistical Analysis

Statistical analyses were performed employing One-way ANOVA followed by the Tukey test/Dunnet test to assess intergroup statistical significance. Additionally, a t-test was utilized for comparing differences between two groups. A total of $n = 6$ samples/group were used for the statistical comparison. The data is expressed as mean $\pm$ standard deviation, with statistical significance deemed for a p value < 0.05.

4.3   Results

4.3.1   Biophysical Characterization of LNPs

Both biotinylated (with PEG-Biotin) LNPs (bLNPs) and non-biotinylated LNPs (i.e., without PEG-Biotin) exhibited strong cationic charges, featuring sizes in the range of 100-150 nm and polydispersity indices below 0.1 **(Figure 37)**. LNPs without PEG-Biotin had an average hydrodynamic diameter of 124.06 ± 17.64 nm, with a polydispersity index of 0.07 ± 0.03. The average zeta potential for non-biotinylatedlated LNPs was 42.96 ± 2.24 mV. In comparison, bLNPs with PEG-Biotin displayed a similar polydispersity index (0.05 ± 0.03) but exhibited a significantly larger hydrodynamic diameter (127.95 ± 10.49 nm, p < 0.0102) compared to their non-biotinylated LNPs. Notably, the zeta potential of bLNPs was significantly reduced, measuring 39.06 ± 5.31 mV (p<0.0001), compared to non-biotinylated LNPs.

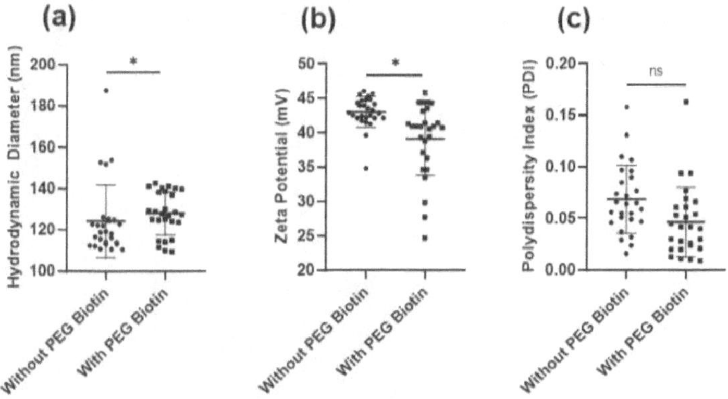

Figure 37: Biophysical properties of LNPs a) Size, b) Charge, c) Polydispersity Index. The data is expressed as the mean ± SD (n=9 readings/formulations per batch). * Indicates statistical significance with p < 0.05

4.3.2 Assessment of LNP Stability in Storage Stability Assessment

The stabilities of both bLNPs and LNPs in storage were evaluated post-formulation, spanning 14 days stored at 4 °C in a water suspension. Through this period, the average hydrodynamic diameter, charge, and polydispersity index exhibited remarkable stability **(Figure 38)**. While there was a noticeable variation in size of LNPs within the initial 24 h, both the LNPs **(Figure 38a, b, c)** and bLNPs **(Figure 38d, e, f)** consistently maintained a size range between 100 nm and 150 nm throughout the observation period. After 14 days, the LNPs were lyophilized and stored at 4°C for future experiments.

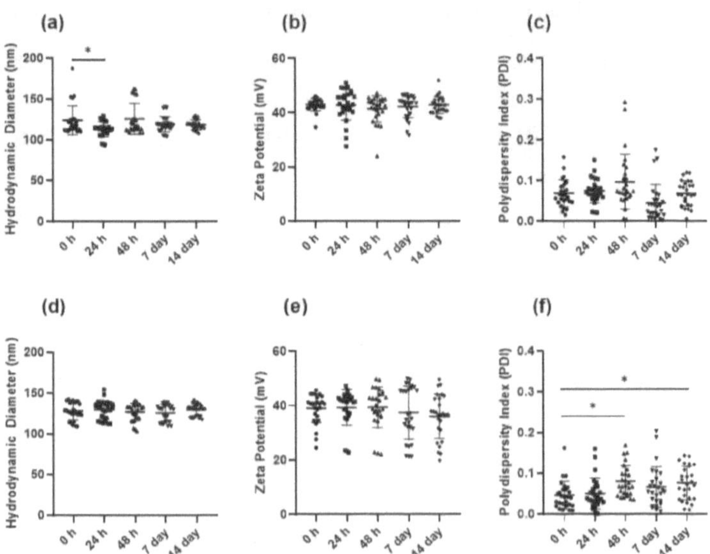

Figure 38: Graph showing the stability of LNPs and bLNPs in storage condition (4 °C). (a, d) shows the stability of hydrodynamic diameter, (b, e) stability of zeta potential, and (c, f) stability in polydispersity index for LNPs without PEG-Biotin and for bLNPs having PEG-Biotin respectively. The data is expressed as the mean ± SD (n = 9). * Indicates statistical significance of differences deemed for $p < 0.05$

4.3.3 Verification of Biotin Conjugation on bLNPs

The conjugation of biotin on bLNPs was confirmed by establishing a standard curve that correlated bLNP concentration with absorbance readings from a biotin quantification assay which was further plotted as bLNP concentration vs quantified biotin (in nmol/μL). The resulting linear curve, with an r-squared value of 0.99 **(Figure 39a, b)**, demonstrated a strong correlation between bLNP concentration and absorbance/Biotin, reaffirming the presence of biotin in our bLNPs. On average, 0.34 nmol of biotin was found per µg of

bLNPs as achieved from **Figure 39b**.

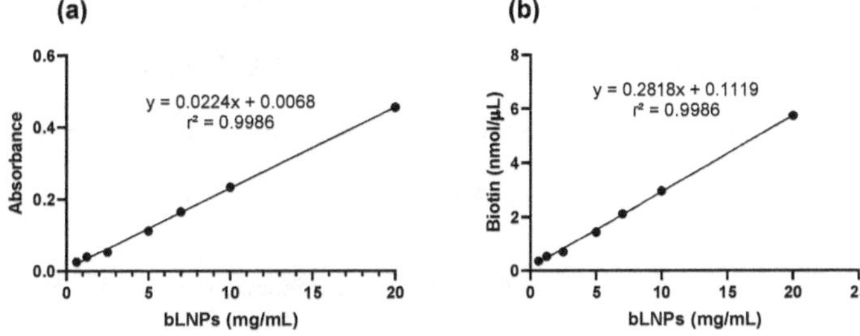

Figure 39: Biotin quantification to determine the degree of biotinylation on bLNPs. Standard curve was established by correlating a) concentration of bLNPs to absorbance readings, b) bLNP concentratiosn to nmol of biotin per microliters of bLNPs, based on the standard curve obtained from the former correlation

4.3.4 Encapsulation Efficiency of SNPs

SNP encapsulation in bLNPs, quantified using a Greiss reagent assay, was found to be

consistent across LNP batches. Encapsulation efficiency was determined to be $52.1 \pm 6.8\%$,

$60.1 \pm 2.0\%$ and $57.0 \pm 6.9\%$ for batches 1, 2 and 3 respectively. (n = 3 replicate

measurements).

4.3.5 In-Vitro SNP Release and Curve Fitting based on Korsmeyer-Peppas Model

Figure 40 shows the profile of *in-vitro* relative release of SNP from bLNPs. The

relative release profiles of SNP from bLNPs, assessed based on the detected nitrite levels

at specified time points, display a biphasic pattern, characterized by an initial burst release

within the first 24 h. This is followed by a slower, sustained release of the drug beyond 24 h with detectable nitrite levels observed even on day 45. The application of the Korsmeyer-Peppas (KP) model to curve-fit our experimental data yielded a remarkable r-squared value of 0.98, indicating an exceptionally close fit of the data. Additionally, the values obtained for k and n as shown in equation 1 were 0.89 and 0.027 respectively. Based on this model, we determined the required concentration of the drug to be loaded into the bLNPs (~0.25 mg/mL) to achieve 100 nM of SNP release was 3.756 µM (1.12 mg/mL) of SNP.

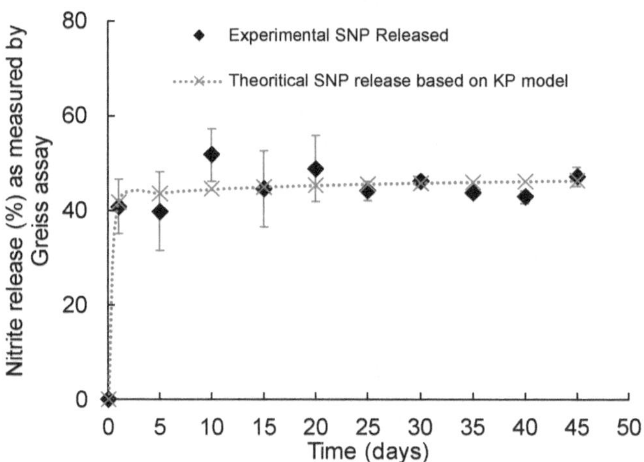

Figure 40: Graph showing the kinetics of relative SNP released, quantified by measuring the corresponding percentage of nitrite release through the Greiss assay. The red dashed line with an 'x' denotes the curve fitting based on the Korsmeyer-Peppas model. The data is expressed as the mean ± standard deviation (SD)

4.3.6 Cytotoxicity Evaluation of bLNPs

We assessed the cytotoxicity of bLNPs in aHASMCs, given the higher positive charge observed in our LNPs, to ensure their compatibility with aHASMCs. The LIVE/DEAD assay revealed significant loss in aHASMC viability when exposed to 1 mg/mL concentration of bLNPs; viability was only 26.75 ± 7.69% **(Figure 41)**. At other doses bLNPs aHASMC viabilities were 89.86 ± 6.18% (p<0.005 vs untreated control), and 92.45 ± 3.16% (p<0.0001 vs untreated control) at 0.5 mg/mL, and 0.1 mg/mL respectively, whereas the viability was not significantly different compared to controls at the 0.25 mg/ mL dose of bLNPs (95.17 ± 1.39%). Across tested bLNP dose range, the overall viability thus decreased by at most 12%.

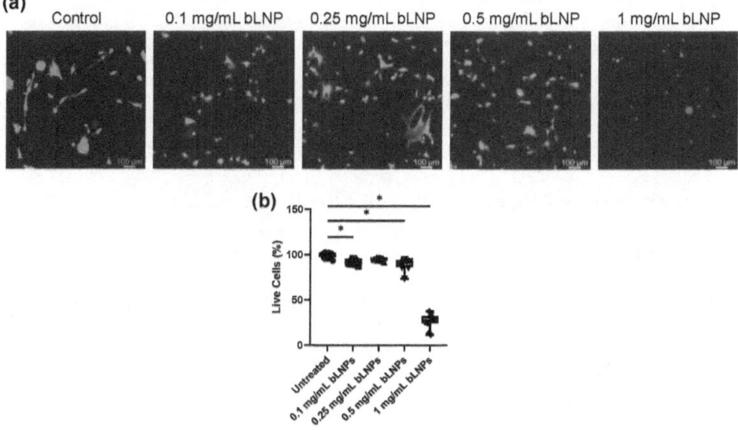

Figure 41: Effects of bLNPs on the viability of aHASMCs as observed in the (a) LIVE/DEAD assay. Live cells are represented in green whereas dead cells are indicated in red. (b) graphical representation of cell viability in percentage based on green signals of live cells normalized to total signal intensity of both green and red. The data is expressed as the mean ± SD (n = 6). * Indicates statistical significance of differences deemed for p < 0.05

4.3.7   Confirming NA-Bridging within LCGs

To verify the Neutravidin (NA)-mediated conjugation of bLNPs onto bPCL for the development of novel LCGs, we utilized fluorescence imaging to illustrate three distinct graft scenarios: PCL+NA488+bLNP, bPCL+NA488+LNP, and bPCL+NA488+bLNP. In the first case, incubating Dylight NA488 with the PCL graft resulted in the lack of NA retention, indicated by the weak green signal of NA in Figure 42**b** and the representative graph in Figure 42**d**. This lack of NA retention indicated the absence of bLNPs conjugation, as evident by the weak red signal of DiR-labeled bLNPs (Figure 42**b, d**). In the second case, incubating Dylight NA-488 with the bPCL graft led to significantly higher green signal retention ($p<0.001$) compared to the PCL+NA488+bLNP group, as depicted in the second row of **Figure 42b** and in the representative graph (**Figure 42d**). However, there was no conjugation of DiR-labeled LNPs in this instance since these LNPs lacked biotin (**Figure 42b, c**). Finally, in the third case, incubating bPCL with Dylight NA-488, followed by incubation with bLNPs, resulted in significantly higher retention of both green signal ($p <0.0001$ compared to the PCL+NA488+bLNP group) and red signal ($p <0.0001$ compared to the PCL+NA488+bLNP and bPCL+NA488+LNP groups), as shown in the third row of **Figure 42b**, and representative graphs shown in **Figure 42(c, d).** This case successfully demonstrated the conjugation of both Dylight NA-488 and bLNPs.

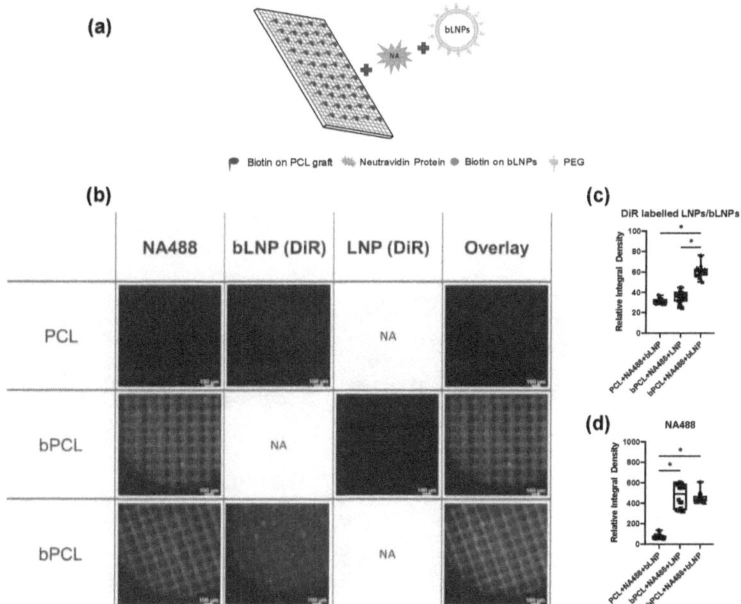

Figure 42: Neutravidin (NA)-mediated conjugation of bLNPs onto bPCL meshes for lipid nanoparticle charged graft (LCGs) development. (a) Illustration of the conjugation process: PCL meshes (with or without biotin) were incubated with Dylight NA488 for 1 h, followed by DiR-labeled LNP (with and without biotin) for 1 h. Conjugation was performed in three different cases: PCL + NA488 + bLNPs, bPCL + NA488 + LNPs, and bPCL + NA488 + bLNPs (b) Fluorescence images of PCL mesh after *in-vitro* conjugation: DyLight NA488 binding to PCL meshes (with or without biotin) in green and LNPs (with and without biotin) conjugation to NA488 in red. (c) Graphs depicting fluorescence intensity of LNPs binding, and (d) NA488 binding. The data is expressed as the mean ± SD (n = 6). * Indicates statistical significance of differences deemed for p < 0.05

4.3.8   Cytotoxicity Assessment of LCGs

The cytotoxicity of LCGs was evaluated in both contact and non-contact cell culture models, revealing a high degree of compatibility with minimal or no cell death. In the contact model **(Figure 43 b, c)**, cell viability was notably high, with values of 93.74 ±

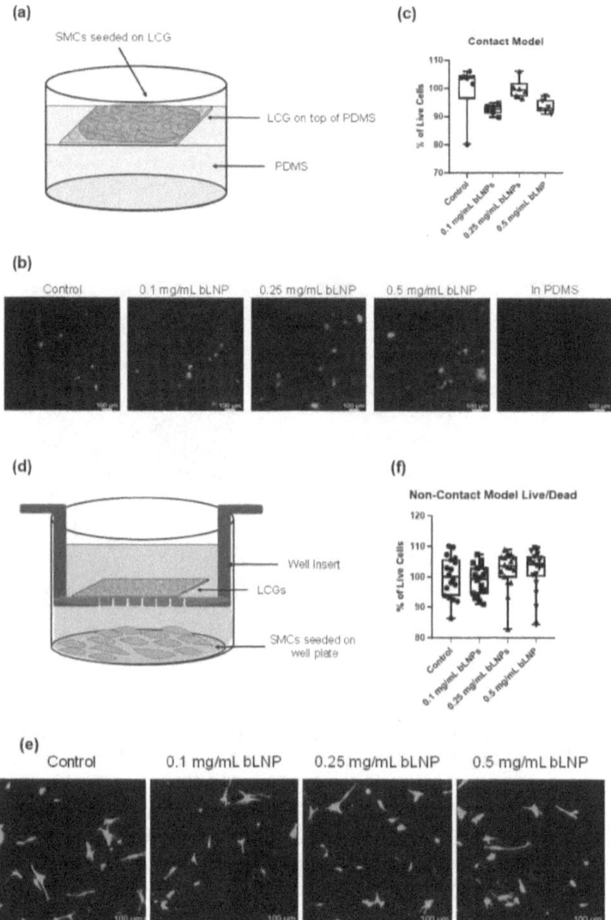

Figure 43: Figure illustrating the cytotoxicity assessment of LCGs using contact and non-contact models. (a, d) Visual depiction of the *in-vitro* exposure methods for the contact and non-contact models, respectively. (b, e) LIVE/DEAD assay images of aHASMCs with live cells in green and dead cells in red for the contact and non-contact models respectively. (c, f) Statistical comparisons represented in graphs based on LIVE/DEAD assay results. The data is expressed as the mean ± SD (n=6 cultures/condition). * Indicates statistical significance of differences deemed for p < 0.05

2.37%, 99.95 ± 3.40%, and 92.57 ± 1.76% observed for cells in contact with LCGs conjugated with 0.5 mg/mL, 0.25 mg/mL, and 0.1 mg/mL of bLNPs, respectively. Similarly, in the non-contact culture model **(Figure 43 e, f)**, slightly higher aHASMC viability were seen with percentages of 102.43 ± 6.75%, 102.44 ± 6.33%, and 98.92 ± 4.94% when treated with LCGs conjugated with 0.5 mg/mL, 0.25 mg/mL, and 0.1 mg/mL of bLNPs,

4.3.9   Gene Expression of Key ECM Homeostasis Proteins

To assess the impact of SNP-releasing LCGs on the gene expression of key ECM homeostasis markers by cultured aHASMCs, RT-PCR was performed for *MMP2*, *TIMP1*, *TIMP2*, *TIMP4*, *COLIIIA1*, *ELN*, and *LOX* **(Figure 44)**. The treatment with SNP LCGs was conducted in a non-contact model to closely mimic physiological relevance, ensuring that if placed periadventitially, the LCGs would not be in direct contact with SMCs. The gene expression study revealed a significant reduction in *MMP2* expression (p<0.001), coupled with an upregulation of its inhibitors *TIMP2* (p<0.05) and *TIMP4* (p<0.05). However, there was no statistically significant difference in *TIMP1* gene expression. Moreover, there was a decrease in *COLIIIA1* gene expression, although it did not reach statistical significance in our analysis. Additionally, SNP LCGs demonstrated a notable upregulation in the gene expression of elastic matrix assembly genes *ELN* (p<0.001) and *LOX* (p<0.001) compared to the control. There was no statistical difference in relative gene expression of aHASMCs between control aHASMC cultures vs aHASMCs treated with blank LCGs.

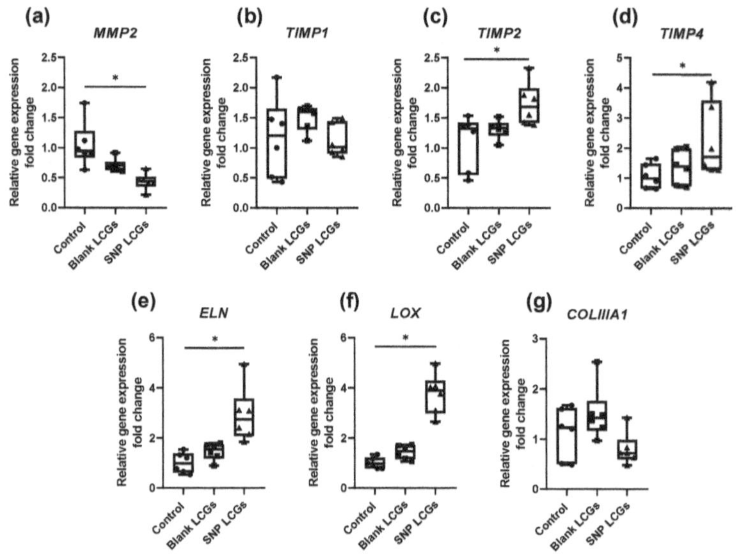

Figure 44: Effect of SNP LCGs on expression of genes for various ECM homeostasis proteins (a) *MMP2*, (b) *TIMP1*, (c) *TIMP2*, (d) *TIMP4*, (e) *ELN*, (f) *LOX*, (g) *COLIIIA1*. The data is expressed as the mean ± SD (n = 6 cultures/condition). * Indicates statistical significance of differences deemed for p < 0.05

4.3.10 Expression of Proteins Critical to Elastic Matrix Homeostasis

The results from our gene expression study were further validated through assessment of protein expression by western blot (WB) analysis (**Figure 45**) and IF imaging. In WB analysis, the protein expression of MMP2 was significantly downregulated (p <0.01 vs. control) following treatment with SNP LCGs. A similar effect was observed in the expression of LOX (p <0.05 vs. controls), which increased with the administration of SNP LCGs. However, no statistical difference was observed in the expression of TIMP4. TIMP1 and TIMP2 remained undetected in our WB analysis.

In our IF studies, there was a significant increase in elastin expression compared to that of both control and blank LCG treatment (**Figure 45** d, e).

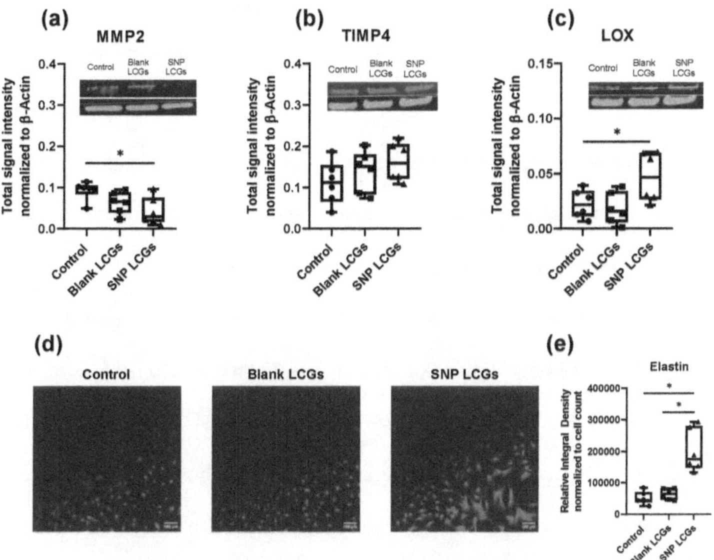

Figure 45: Effects of SNP LCGs on ECM homeostasis proteins as determined by WB analysis. (a-c) The total signal intensity of each analyzed proteins normalized to β-actin expression with their respective WB gel blots. (d) Immunofluorescence (IF) based staining of newly formed elastin by aHASMCs when treated with SNP LCGs in non-contact model. Red signal represents elastin and blue represents nuclei. (e) Representative statistical comparison of elastin expression as seen in IF. The data is expressed as the mean ± SD (n = 6). * Indicates statistical significance of differences deemed for p < 0.05

4.3.11 Decellularization and Controlled Elastic Matrix Disruption in PCA

Decellularization was carried out on three batches of porcine carotid arteries, with each batch including six images representing the top, middle, and bottom sections. This process involved an initial 24 h incubation in 0.5% v/v Triton-X, followed by subsequent incubations for 24, 36, 48, and 72 h in 0.25% v/v SDS **(Figure 46a, b, c)**. The histological analysis revealed a decreased number of residual cells after Triton-X incubation resulting in drop of cell density to $76.5 \pm 2.85\%$. Subsequent incubations in SDS for 24 h, 36 h, 48 h, and 72 h resulted in further reductions, yielding $53.62 \pm 3.23\%$, $33.02 \pm 2.29\%$, $10.91 \pm 2.00\%$, and $3.17 \pm 1.98\%$, respectively. It's worth mentioning that beyond 36 h of SDS decellularization, there was an extremely low presence of single DAPI-stained nuclei. The cell nuclei appeared to disintegrate, leading to the dispersion of the blue signal. Additionally, a substantial decrease in elastic matrix fluorescence intensity was also observed after each decellularization step, with residual elastin percentages of $81.77 \pm 6.74\%$ after 24 h of Triton-X exposure, and $77.06 \pm 6.05\%$, $76.50 \pm 6.78\%$, $71.08 \pm 6.82\%$, and $68.97 \pm 6.86\%$ following 24 h, 36 h, 48 h, and 72 h of SDS incubation. Statistical analysis showed significant differences in total cell density among the groups ($p < 0.0001$), except for the comparison between 48 h SDS and 72 h SDS, which had a significance level of $p < 0.5$. Similarly, there was a significant reduction in relative residual elastin fluorescence intensity at each decellularization time point when compared to the native control (Native vs. Triton X; $p < 0.05$, Native vs. 24 h SDS and Native vs. 36 h SDS; $p < 0.005$, and Native vs. 48 h SDS, Native vs. 72 h SDS; $p < 0.0001$).

Furthermore, the elastase infusion caused significant damage to the ECM elastin when compared to the non-decellularized native PCA control and decellularized PCA (24 h in Triton X and 36 h in SDS) that was not subjected to elastic matrix degradation **(Figure 46d, e)**. The overall percentage of the residual elastic matrix exhibited a significant decrease, reducing from 100% in the native controls (no decellularization, no elastase incubation) to $76.50 \pm 6.78\%$ ($p < 0.005$) in decellularized PCAs, and to $61.32 \pm 6.66\%$ (p

<0.0001), 51.26 ± 6.35% (p<0.0001), and 32.80 ± 5.99% (p <0.0001) after 1 h, 2 h, and 3

h of incubation with 96 units of elastase.

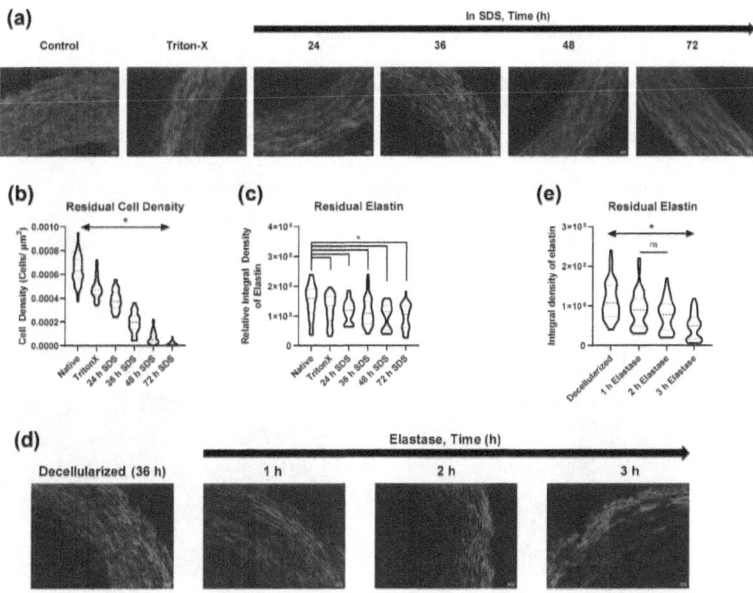

Figure 46: Fluorescence images illustrating the histological staining of porcine
carotid arteries (PCA). (a) Histological images displaying native control and
decellularized PCAs following various decellularization durations. (b, c) Violin plots
showing statistical analysis of residual cell density and remaining elastin content at
different decellularization time points. (d) Histological images comparing decellularized
PCA (36 h) to elastic matrix damage at various elastase incubation durations (94
units/mL). (e) Statistical evaluation of elastase impact on elastin retention. The red signal
corresponds to elastin staining using Pontamine Sky Blue, while the blue signals indicate
nuclei stained with DAPI. The data is expressed as the mean ± SD (n = 54
images/condition). * Indicates statistical significance of differences deemed for p < 0.05

4.3.12 Assessment of Cytocompatibility of SNP-bLNPs on aHASMCs Seeded on Decellularized, Matrix-Disrupted PCA

The porcine carotid artery exhibited excellent compatibility when recellularized with aHASMCs, as indicated by a cell viability of $89.75 \pm 5.43\%$ after 72 h of culture. In **Figure 12**, there is minimal presence of the red signal, which is associated with Ethidium bromide staining for dead cells. The 3D stacked images correspond to our 2D LIVE/DEAD assay results, with a significant portion of the 3D construct displaying a green signal and only a small fraction exhibiting the red signal.

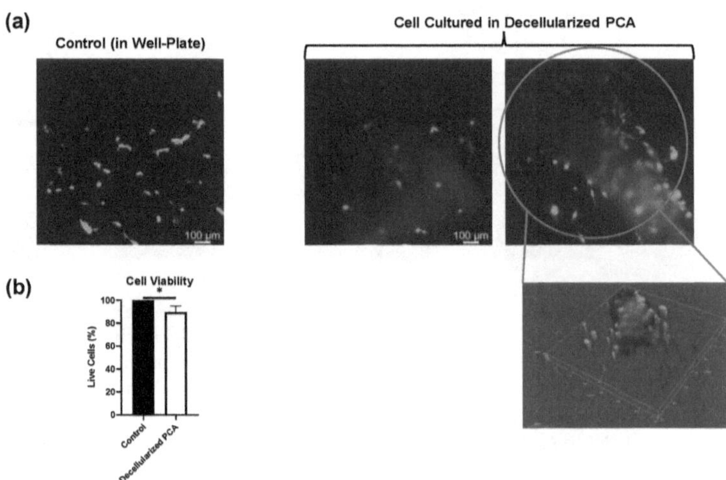

Figure 47: LIVE/DEAD assay demonstrating aHASMC cytocompatibility after 72 h of culture on dPCA. (a) Side-by-side comparison of cell fluorescence images between control and decellularized PCA (24 h in Triton X-100 and 36 h in SDS followed by a 2 h of incubation with elastase) along with their respective 3D images captured via z-stacking. The data is expressed as the mean $\pm$ SD (n = 6). * Indicates statistical significance with $p < 0.05$

4.3.13 Expression of ECM Homeostasis Proteins on Recellularized PCA

The expression of MMP2 in rPCAs significantly decreased when treated with SNP LCGs compared to the control and blank LCGs (p<0.01) **(Figure 48a,b)**. In contrast, TIMP2, an immediate inhibitor of MMP2, exhibited a significant increase with SNP LCGs treatment (p<0.001) **(Figure 48a,c)** . Additionally, the expression of elastin was significantly upregulated with SNP treatment (p<0.001) compared to both control and blank LCGs**(Figure 48a,d)**. No significant difference was observed between control rPCAs and those treated with blank LCGs alone in any cases.

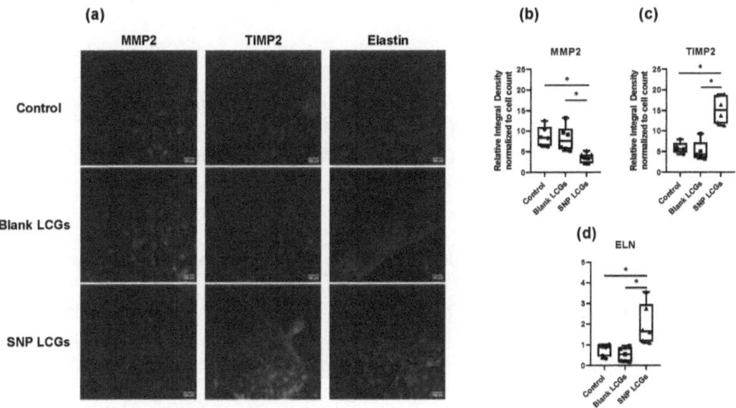

Figure 48: IF based demonstration of expression of ECM homeostasis proteins in porcine carotid artery (rPCA) recellularized with aHASMCs when treated with SNP LCGs for 7 days in non-contact mode. The data is expressed as the mean ± SD (n=6). * Indicates statistical significance of differences deemed for p < 0.05

4.4   Discussion

AAAs pose a severe threat to the elderly population, afflicting 6-9% of this demographic with a devastating mortality rate exceeding 90% upon rupture[73]. Although smaller AAAs can be conservatively managed through continuous monitoring and risk factor control (e.g., smoking, hypertension, low-fat diet etc.), the morbidity and mortality associated with ruptured AAAs continue to be high. Progressive growth of AAAs is linked to the gradual deterioration of the structural integrity of the aorta wall, which in turn is critically dependent on the intricate assembly, crosslinking, organization, and alignment of elastic and collagen fibers within the wall ECM[261,276]. These structures provide strength, and stretch and recoil abilities to the AAA wall, which diminishes as the elastic matrix degrades, mainly due to chronic local overexpression of MMP s (specifically MMP2 and MMP9) triggered by injury-induced inflammation and/or oxidative stress[109,277]. Presently, the standard of care involves surgeries for large pre-rupture stage AAAs, yet they fail to effectively halt or slow the progression of aneurysms along the aortic wall due to lack of control in the persisting inflammation, VSMCs degradation, proteolytic degradation, and endothelial dysfunction. Therefore, there is an urgent need for alternative, less invasive treatments targeting AAA pathophysiology that can restore wall homeostasis as an outcome. NO, primarily produced by ECs, has been previously shown to positively regulate vascular tone, inflammation, VSMCs phenotypic modulation, angiogenesis, platelet activation, leukocyte adhesion and proteolytic (MMPs) and anti-proteolytic (TIMPs) parameters of vascular walls[46]. Our previous study also highlights the significant role of the NO donor drug, SNP, in inhibiting proteolytic enzymes like MMP2, often linked with AAAs, while also promoting elastic matrix assembly, crosslinking, and maturation through MAPK pathway inhibition[260]. Yet, the short half-life of NO severely limits its efficacy. The administration of oral drugs also faces biological and biochemical barriers along the gastrointestinal tract, ultimately leading to drug degradation and diminishing their bioavailability to the tissue[178,278]. Towards addressing these limitations, our current study sought to develop lipid nanoparticle charged grafts (LCGs) by conjugating bLNPs to bPCL meshes using neutravidin (NA) bridging. This approach may enable localized SNP delivery to SMCs within the aortal medial layer, to stimulate elastic matrix assembly and anti-proteolytic effects.

To prepare bLNPs, we used DOTAP as the main cationic component to impart a positive surface charge. Notably, the biodegradable ester linker in DOTAP is less toxic than other lipid components[279]. To improve the functional properties and safety of these LNPs, we conjugated them with 40% w/w of DSPE PEG-Biotin; this would serve to leverage the properties of PEG in enhancing circulation time (if applicable), preventing self-aggregation, and reducing cytotoxicity, and that of the biotin component in enabling ligand-receptor-mediated targeting[279,280]. Our study demonstrated significant cytocompatibility of the bLNPs, even at high concentrations of 0.5 mg/mL, with less than ~12% cell death in cultures of aHASMC isolated from patients with rupture-stage AAAs **(Figure 41)**. The incorporation of phospholipids and PEG also confers hydrophobic and hydrophilic properties respectively to bLNPs, rendering them versatile for drug delivery, gene transfection, and vaccine delivery[281]. Additionally, DSPE PEG-Biotin fortifies the bLNPs bilayer, making it more resistant to enzymatic degradation and enabling the design of novel LCGs based on the robust interactions between biotin and neutravidin[282,283].

Biophysical characterization revealed an increase in size of the bLNPs, likely due to the additional phospholipid component incorporated within these bLNPs, while the decrease in charge can be attributed to the anionic PEG component of DSPE PEG-Biotin, which masks the cationic charge, as reported in other previous studies[264,284]. Furthermore, PEG provides steric shielding to inhibit aggregation, as evident by our very low PDI values **(Figure 37c),** and significantly interactions with proteins and proteases to prevent surface fouling of the bLNPs[285]. This is corroborated by our stability test, where bLNPs stored as a suspension at 4 °C for 14 days showed no significant increase in the size and in the PDI, indicating that the LNPs (with and without biotin) remained homogeneously monodispersed within the size range of 100-150 nm and did not fuse or aggregate **(Figure 38)**. Additionally, the observed SNP encapsulation efficiency in bLNPs measured as 56.41 ± 2.80% (mean ± SD), aligns with values reported for other drugs, highlighting suitability for therapeutic application[286,287]. Our findings suggest that the presence of cationic excipients may be a prerequisite for achieving higher encapsulation efficiency of SNP, which warrants further validation in follow-up studies. The release profile of SNP was characterized by an initial rapid burst release within the first 24 h, likely resulting from the immediate release of loosely encapsulated or surface-entrapped drugs, followed by a stable, continuous release **(Figure 40)**. This behavior can be attributed to SNP's stability as an NO donor, as well as the stability of LNPs conferred by cholesterol and DOPE[175,288]. The incorporation of cholesterol in bLNPs likely contributed to the prolonged release observed in our experiments. Previous studies have demonstrated that cholesterol enhances the packing of phospholipid molecules, decreasing bilayer permeability and modifying intravesicular fluidity which can collectively increase rigidity, to slow release[288-291]. Our release kinetic model, based on the KP model's equation, yielded a correlation coefficient of 0.98 demonstrating a remarkable fit of experimental data to theoretical release, and the calculated transport exponent value of n = 0.027 which is less than ~0.5 indicates that diffusion is the primary mechanism driving SNP release[289]. Additionally, the lower drug transport constant (k = 0.89) value, which is less than 1, indicates that drug transport from the bLNPs occurs at a notably slower rate. This observation aligns with the gradual increase in the detected nitrite percentage, indicating sustained release of SNP from bLNPs (**Figure 40**) [292]. One limitation of our SNP release kinetics assessment is that our experiments exclusively capture the relative release of SNP in relation to nitrite detected at specified time points. Both NO and nitrite, having short half-lives, swiftly oxidize to nitrate[293]. To provide a more precise understanding of the absolute release amounts and kinetics of SNP, future investigations should employ a more accurate detection method. This would involve the cumulative measurement of NO, nitrite, and nitrate at these specified time points, offering a comprehensive perspective on SNP release. However, our results indicate SNP release over a 45-day period, as suggested by the detected nitrite percentage. The observed gradual increase in released nitrite percentage over time from bLNPs, with no additional nitrite sources other than SNP, suggests the potential for sustained release over week.

In this study, we employed bLNPs as a simplified model nanocarrier. This choice allowed us to concentrate on their specific interactions crucial for LCG development. For this, we utilized biotin-neutravidin as a well-established pair due to their strong and clearly understood binding affinity[283]. Neutravidin, a de-glycosylated form of avidin that contains four identical subunits, was preferred for its robust binding to biotin without any non-specific interactions[294]. One significant advantage of the biotin-neutravidin-biotin interaction employed in LCG formation is its high affinity, which remains stable against various challenges, including manipulation, exposure to proteolytic enzymes, changes in temperature and pH, and exposure to harsh organic and denaturing reagents[295]. This interaction has found applications in tissue engineering and regeneration, particularly in enhancing bone tissue engineering thereby exhibiting its potential to be used in several other tissue engineering applications[296]. The successful biotinylation of bLNPs, as shown by the calibration curve between bLNP concentration and absorbance or biotin per μg of bLNPs in **Figure 39**, provides evidence for improved bLNP stability. The prolonged stability of bLNPs modified with biotinylated PEG can be attributed to their ability to attach to neutravidin-conjugated biotinylated PCL meshes while resisting nonspecific binding to serum proteins or opsonins[297]. The formation of LCGs by conjugating bLNPs to the 3D-printed bPCL by sandwich biotin-neutravidin-biotin binding can be extended in the future conjugating biotinylated NPs, biotinylated antibodies, or penetrating peptides etc., as may be reqired. In this particular study, we confirm the successful conjugation of bLNPs onto bPCL meshes, as depicted in **Figure 42**. The increased fluorescence intensity of both DiR-labeled bLNPs and Dylight NA 488 in case of bLNP+NA488+bPCL demonstrates that the conjugation was indeed facilitated by the NA bridge, as expected. This research presents a valuable strategy for functionalizing LNPs, improving their potential as drug carriers, and expanding their possible applications, including diagnostic as well as therapeutic application for biomimetic studies in various diseases.

LCGs showed remarkable cytocompatibility when tested on cultured aHASMCs in both non-contact and contact models. In the contact model, where aHASMCs were directly seeded onto LCGs, they adhered and gradually covered the LCGs' scaffold surface within

72 h **(Figure 43)**. Notably, the standard PCL scaffold, known for its hydrophobic nature, typically exhibits lower cell attachment capabilities. However, in the case of our LCGs primarily composed of PCL, the enhanced cell attachment can be attributed to the biotin-neutravidin groups[298]. Numerous studies have highlighted the strong affinity of biotin-avidin conjugates, which significantly improve cell attachment on biotin-avidin-treated nanofibrous matrices, such as those in our LCGs. Our finding is in line with previous research[298,299]. In fact, it has been suggested that the avidin-biotin system can increase cell adhesion strength by a factor of 2-3 compared to the integrin-serum protein system[300]. A similar positive effect on aHASMC viability was observed when the cells were exposed to the LCGs in a non-contact model over the same time period, demonstrating high cytocompatibility and low toxicity of the grafts. Since the non-contact model closely simulates the physiological conditions for potential future applications, which is expected to involve wrapping of the LCG around the AAA wall to periadventitially deliver the SNP, we opted to proceed with this non-contact model. It is important to note that being embedded in the medial layer of the aorta wall, the aneurysmal SMCs would not naturally come into contact with the periadventitially-placed LCGs.

Prior to aHASMCs treatment with SNP-releasing LCGs, we determined the total drug loading levels within the bLNPs, necessary to achieve SNP release at a steady state concentration of 100 nM, as this concentration was identified in our SNP dosing studies (Chapter III) as optimal for stimulating elastic matrix neoassembly[260]. The KP model, adopted in previous studies on liposome drug release kinetics[301], predicted an SNP loading concentration of 3.76 μM (~1.12 μg/mL) within the bLNPs as necessary in preparing SNP LCGs. Afterwards, to investigate the efficacy of LCGs in regenerative repair of AAAs, we performed experiments examining their impact on protein and gene expression in *in-vitro* aHASMC cultures. To achieve this, we formulated LCGs conjugating 0.25 mg/mL of bLNPs loaded with SNP onto the bPCL meshes using NA bridging as described earlier and treated aHASMCs with SNP LCGs in a non-contact way. Our *in-vitro* evaluation of proteins related to elastic matrix homeostasis revealed a significant reduction in MMP2 (**Figure 44a,** and **Figure 45a**) when treated with SNP LCGs. This observation aligned with an increase in the gene and protein expression of MMP2 inhibitors, particularly TIMP2 and TIMP4 (**Figure 44c, d**). Additionally, we noted elevated expression levels of matrix assembly proteins, specifically ELN (**Figure 44e and Figure 45d,e**) and LOX (**Figure 44f and Figure 45c**). NO, despite being relatively unreactive, works via two ways: a) at higher concentrations, it reacts with oxygen or superoxides to generate inflammatory reactive nitrogen species (RNS) to trigger cellular stress and activate stress-activated pathways; b) at lower concentrations, it interacts with metal complexes such as iron-binding proteins of oxyhemoglobin, to activate sGC-cGMP and other intricate pathways that inhibit proteolytic enzymes such as MMP2 and MMP9[220,302,303]. In our study, the release of NO from a sub-IC50 dose of SNP may thus explain the inhibition of MMPs and the upregulation of TIMPs. We observed a similar outcome when LCGs were utilized in an *ex-vivo* rPCA AAA model. In this study, there was a noteworthy decrease in MMP2 (**Figure 48a, b**) expression and a concurrent increase in both TIMP2 (**Figure 48a, c**), and elastin expression, as confirmed by our immunofluorescence study (**Figure 48a, d**). This may likely be related to the evident fact that NO inhibit MAPK proteins (such as ERK and JNK), which serve as upstream regulators of MMP expression in AAAs[260]. Likely, a similar effect might be possible in our study and requires further validation with complex biochemical analysis and TEM studies. This NO-driven activation is crucial for maintaining ECM homeostasis, vascular tone, and cellular functions. Interestingly, our results contrast with findings from various other studies, where NO is described as an activator of MMPs and a key contributor to the pathogenesis of other diseases such as cancers[304,305]. These varying observations may stem from differences in experimental conditions, drug concentrations, and specific disease contexts. Nonetheless, our study highlights the potential of SNP-loaded LCGs in promoting elastic matrix repair and supporting ECM homeostasis in the context of AAAs.

In addition to the evidence supporting the effectiveness of LCGs in stimulating elastic matrix neoassembly and anti-proteolytic effects by aneurysmal SMCs, this study has unveiled several other key findings. Firstly, we devised a decellularization strategy for porcine carotid arteries using a combination of low-concentration Triton X-100 and SDS. Our results demonstrated that the removal of cells and nuclear materials begin within 24 h, and the extent of removal was directly linked to the incubation times **(Figure 46a, b)**[306]. However, a detailed quantitative analysis of DNA in each of these dPCAs would shed more light into the decellularization efficiency of this decellularization technique. Moreover, the decellularization process seemed to lead to the loss of the elastin density over time**(Figure 46a, c)**, likely due to the disruption of elastin's disulfide bonds by these detergents, which is consistent with findings from other studies[307]. Furthermore, to create a physiologically relevant *ex-vivo* AAA model, we exposed our decellularized porcine carotid arteries (dPCA) to elastase, inducing elastic matrix damage. At the strength and dose utilized, elastase rapidly degraded elastin within one h, with more pronounced damage observed with longer incubation times **(Figure 46d, e)**. This method provides an excellent model for

164

studying matrix degradation, as observed in aging, atherosclerosis, and AAAs, contributing to a better understanding of cell-cell and cell-matrix interactions in 3D environment. Additionally, the dPCA demonstrated impressive cytocompatibility by supporting the survival and growth of aHASMCs during the 72 h culture period as shown in the LIVE/DEAD assay result **(Figure 12)**. These results concur with previously published findings showing successful recellularization of PCAs with SMCs and human umblical vein endothelial cells (HUVECs) under static culture condition[308]. The favorable seeding outcome and lack of toxicity can be attributed to the thorough washing of the dPCA for 48 h in DI water after decellularization, followed by an additional ethanol wash, all without disrupting ECM components, which helped in washing off all the residual detergent concentrations[309].

In conclusion, the findings of this study shed light on the promising potential of LCGs for in situ regenerative repair of AAAs. The remarkable cytocompatibility and encouraging results in both *in-vitro* and *ex-vivo* models suggest that LCGs, specifically those conjugated with biotin-Neutravidin interaction and loaded with SNP, hold great promise in promoting elastic matrix repair and maintaining ECM homeostasis.

In summary, LCGs significantly downregulated MMP2, and upregulated proteins key to ECM homeostasis and vascular health such as elastin, LOX, TIMP2, and TIMP4. These findings are further substantiated by the positive outcomes in *ex-vivo* dPCA AAA model when recellularized with aHASMCs, as they exhibited cytocompatibility and allowed cell growth, and demonstrated evidence of anti-proteolysis (MMP2 downregulation) and elastic matrix neoassembly (upregulated elastin). Moreover, the sustained release behavior of SNP from the LCGs, demonstrated through the Korsmeyer-Peppas model, highlights the potential for controlled and long-lasting therapeutic delivery. The significant reduction in MMP2, a major contributor to AAA development, offers promise in slowing disease progression. While the role of NO in regulating ECM homeostasis has been a subject of debate, our results align with studies indicating its inhibitory effect on proteolytic enzymes, such as MMP2, while promoting elastic matrix assembly. By addressing the short half-life of NO through the use of LCGs, we have the opportunity to achieve more sustained and effective ECM repair. Overall, this study introduces a novel strategy for LCG development, successfully conjugating bLNPs onto bPCL meshes to create an efficient functional nanodrug conjugates for localized SNP delivery. Our findings reveal that LCGs are cytocompatible, facilitating cell attachment despite the hydrophobic nature of PCL, and offer sustained SNP release over 45 days, which stimulates the expression of genes and proteins associated with elastin homeostasis. These results hold promise for the continued development and testing of LCGs to assess their therapeutic efficacy in enhancing elastic matrix homeostasis within an aneurysmal *in-vivo* tissue environment. LCGs have shown great potential in enhancing elastic matrix repair and have far-reaching implications in the development of therapeutic strategies for AAAs. While further research and clinical studies are needed, the results presented here mark a significant step towards more effective treatments for this life-threatening condition and offer new insights into the dynamic role of NO in maintaining vascular health and ECM homeostasis.

CHAPTER V: Conclusion and Future Directions

5.1   Overall Conclusion

The first aim of this book was to characterize and validate anti-proteolytic and pro-elastogenic benefits of the NO donor compound, Sodium Nitroprusside (SNP). The selection of SNP was based on three key criteria: a) ability to release NO in a stable manner, b) release NO at a suitable rate, and c) prior FDA approval for clinical use as a drug to treat hypertension. After roughly sketching our experimental plan for utilizing SNP to assess its feasibility in the regenerative repair of AAAs, we delved into its potential benefits on in vitro aHASMCs cultures. This exploration aimed to understand its reparative properties in terms of ECM homeostasis, particularly its role in enhancing elastic matrix synthesis, assembly, and maturation. Simultaneously, we investigated its capacity to inhibit proteolytic MMPs, which play a crucial role in elastic matrix degradation within the AAA wall. In pursuit of these objectives, we initially established a non-cytotoxic dosing regimen based on the IC50 (50% inhibitory concentration on cell survival) value of SNP. In parallel to this experiment, we also examined the impact of cytokine exposure on aHASMCs' ability to exhibit more severe disease-like phenotypes, a key feature of AAAs. This approach aimed to replicate chronic inflammatory phenotypes in cultured conditions, thereby exaggerating the disease state to validate our hypothesis that SNP, as a NO donor, could serve as an effective treatment strategy even at maximal disease state. This successfully demonstrated its capability to enhance elastic matrix regeneration under these chronic circumstances. Some key findings of this book are discussed below.

5.1.1   Impact of Exogenous SNP on aHASMCs

The first aim of this book successfully highlighted the significant impact of exogenous sodium nitroprusside (SNP), a NO donor, on the phenotypic behavior of aHASMCs. The administration of SNP induced a transition toward contractile-like phenotypes. This occured despite aHASMCs being in a resting phase, evidenced by a non-proliferative cellular state, consistent end-stage SMC contractile marker expressions (e.g., no change in CNN and SMTN gene expression), and a reduction in cellular forces (e.g., including adhesion force, tether force, and Young's modulus). Moreover, the optimal concentration of 100 nM SNP, based on our assessment of gene and protein expressions by the aHASMCs over a range of tested SNP doses, exhibited a robust inhibitory effect of SNP on MMP2 expression, with concurrent upregulation of TIMPs, especially TIMP2 and TIMP4. This led to an enhanced TIMPs to MMP2 ratio, evocative of improved ECM stability. The stimulated assembly of elastic fibers by aHASMCs as evidenced by TEM and elevated elastin and lysyl oxidase (LOX) expressions (both genes and protein), coupled with reduced collagen production, contributed to an improved elastin to collagen ratio. This is an important finding because an appropriate ratio of elastin to collagen ensures adequate compliance of the aorta wall restoring their stretch and recoil properties.

Beyond their implications for AAA treatment, these findings open avenues for alternative applications. The ability of SNP to modulate cellular phenotypes and enhance ECM homeostasis suggests its potential in diverse therapeutic contexts, such as tissue engineering, regenerative medicine, and interventions targeting pathological conditions characterized by ECM dysregulation. Examples of such conditions encompass connective tissue disorders (e.g., Ehlers-Danlos Syndrome), chronic obstructive pulmonary disease (e.g., Emphysema), atherosclerosis, Marfan syndrome, pelvic organ prolapse, among others, all of which exhibit chronic proteolytic degradation of elastic matrix or loss in elastic matrix regenerative abilities. This research not only furthers our understanding of SNP's impact on aHASMCs but also underscores its versatility as a potential therapeutic agent with broad applications in the realm of biomedical research and clinical interventions.

5.1.2 Addressing Pharmacokinetic Challenges

In addressing the challenges posed by uncertain pharmacokinetics during exogenous/oral drug administration, arising from biological and biochemical barriers, such as enzymes (e.g., lipase) and acids (e.g., HCL), we introduced a novel approach. Our focus was on developing functional nanodrug conjugates, referred to as lipid nanoparticle charged grafts (LCGs). We employed the robust biotin-neutravidin binding system to successfully conjugate biotinylated LNPs encapsulated with required concentrations of SNP onto biotinylated PCL meshes. This design was specifically tailored for its potential future use as a drug-eluting vascular graft intended for periadventitial placement in the treatment of AAAs. LCGs offer dual benefits: providing mechanical support to the vascular wall during their frequent stretch and recoil, safeguarding against ruptures, and delivering controlled release of the active ingredient (e.g., SNP) for elastic matrix regeneration and MMP inhibition.

5.1.3   Evaluation of SNP-Releasing LCGs

Our investigation was aimed to assess the efficacy of SNP-eluting LCGs in impeding aneurysm formation, conducted both in vitro and *ex-vivo* in our second and third aim of this book. First, we evaluated SNP LCGs efficacy, gauging their capacity to inhibit AAAs by MMP inhibition and facilitating de novo elastic matrix regeneration. Additionally, a proof-of-concept study explored the viability of a recellularized porcine carotid artery, first decellularized to remove cells and retain the ECM, and lastly inducing elastic matrix damage, as an elastase-induced AAA model. The study was extended to investigate SNP LCGs' feasibility in regenerative repair of the elastic matrix within AAA walls.

Our findings indicate that bLNPs, produced through thin film hydration techniques and extrusion, maintain a hydrodynamic size of 100-150 nm. With a cationic charge of approximately +39 mV, they prove non-cytotoxic to primary diseased aHASMCs, even at concentrations as high as 0.5 mg/mL. Successful encapsulation of SNP in bLNPs, achieving an encapsulation efficiency of ~56% (consistently reproducible across batches), affirms a sustained release of SNP over 45 days through a diffusion mechanism. This holds particular significance, as it extends the drug-eluting half-life, potentially reducing the need for frequent surgical interventions associated with drug-graft replacements. Furthermore, our study confirms that LCGs feature a neutravidin bridge forming a sandwiched conjugation of bLNPs onto bPCL meshes and demonstrated higher aHASMCs cytocompatibility in both contact and non-contact model as shown by our viability study (showing <12% cell death). Beyond the realm of AAAs, the findings suggest that bLNPs hold considerable promise as a platform for drug delivery, gene transfection, and vaccine delivery, owing to their hydrophilic-hydrophobic balance and stability. The successful conjugation of bLNPs onto biotinylated polymer meshes opens avenues for diverse applications in tissue engineering and regenerative medicine and may also serves as an innovative scaffold or platform for 3D culture disease models for drug screening. The sustained release behavior and stability of bLNPs present a valuable proposition for reducing the need for frequent surgical interventions in drug eluting graft replacements.

5.1.4   Utilization of SNP LCGs in In-vitro and Ex-vivo Assessments

The utilization of SNP LCGs in *in-vitro* assessments with aHASMCs, gauging their impact on elastic matrix homeostasis through the inhibition of MMPs, upregulation of TIMPs, and increased expression of matrix assembly proteins like LOX and elastin, underscores their potential for therapeutic applications. The significant reduction in gene and protein expressions of MMPs, particularly MMP2, and the concurrent elevation of LOX, elastin, and MMP inhibitors (TIMPs), highlight the noteworthy ability of SNP LCGs to restore ECM homeostasis. Building on our prior research, which demonstrated SNP's capacity to promote a contractile subpopulation of SMCs in culture, our current *in-vitro* evaluations may feature similar outcomes in terms of phenotypic modulation of aHASMCs which could be a potential topic of exploration in future.

Furthermore, the outcomes observed in the *ex-vivo* disease model, utilizing the elastic matrix-degraded decellularized porcine carotid artery, closely mirrored the *in-vitro* results. This particular aim was designed to present a limited proof-of-concept study, demonstrating the feasibility of LCGs as potential SNP-eluting grafts for therapeutic applications. Our focus was specifically on assessing the ability of SNP LCGs to promote elastic matrix regeneration, as indicated by elastin expression, and to inhibit proteolysis, as indicated by MMP2 and TIMP2 expression. Initially, we successfully re-cellularized the decellularized porcine carotid artery (dPCA) with aHASMCs, confirming the cytocompatibility of these re-cellularized structures for 3D aHASMC culture through our LIVE/DEAD assay results. Subsequently, in a non-contact model, we introduced SNP LCGs to evaluate their efficacy on recellularized PCAs. Remarkably, our findings demonstrated that SNP LCG treatment significantly reduced MMP2 protein expression, showing a positive correlation with the upregulation of TIMP2 and elastin expression. This discovery is particularly exciting as it provides evidence that SNP LCGs contribute to improving ECM homeostasis in both *in-vitro* and *ex-vivo* AAA models, especially when employed as a non-contact treatment option.

This research not only contributes to our understanding of nanocarrier systems for targeted drug delivery but also paves the way for broader applications in the field of biomedical engineering. The potential use of bLNPs in diverse therapeutic contexts, coupled with their stability and controlled release characteristics, suggests a promising future for this technology in enhancing both diagnostic and therapeutic approaches. As we continue to unravel the multifaceted capabilities of bLNPs, their role in advancing personalized medicine and addressing various medical challenges becomes increasingly evident, marking a significant stride towards the realization of innovative and effective biomedical solutions. In conclusion, our comprehensive investigation into the therapeutic potential of SNP LCGs extend beyond aortic aneurysms, making them a valuable and innovative tool in the broader landscape of biomedical solutions.

5.2   Limitations of the study

Although the results of this study were in accordance with our hypothesis, there were some limitations which are listed below:

1.   The use of SNP as a NO donor introduces cytotoxicity concerns due to its simultaneous release of cyanide. This limitation restricts the exploration of higher doses in experiments, as elevated levels could induce cytokine release syndrome and cellular damage.

2.   The study primarily relies on standalone cultures of aHASMCs. In reality, AAAs involve diverse cell types, including macrophages, fibroblasts, and endothelial cells. To enhance clinical relevance, future research should incorporate coculture systems that mimic the intricate cellular crosstalk within the AAA wall milieu.

3.   The book lacks a thorough examination of responses by cells derived from multiple AAA patients. Focusing mostly on a single patient-derived cell type restricts the ability to predict outcomes in the diverse context of individual patient variability.

4.   Reliance on simplified models, such as 2D cell cultures and decellularized porcine carotid arteries, may oversimplify the complex in vivo environment. The findings might not fully represent the intricate interactions and responses within a living organism regulated by spectrum of cells .

5.   Although the study establishes an optimal concentration of 100 nM SNP, a wider dose study is necessary. This would provide a more nuanced understanding of dose-dependent effects and potential variations in outcomes.

6. While the study investigates gene expression of smooth muscle cell (SMC) phenotypic markers, it does not specifically examine their protein expression. Protein-level analysis is crucial for a comprehensive understanding of cellular responses.

7. The relatively lower protein production by aHASMC cultures poses challenges in detecting the expression of key extracellular matrix (ECM) proteins, such as TIMP1 and TIMP2, in Western blotting despite their apparent expression in immunofluorescence studies.

8. Gene expression measurements in the first aim, based on pooled samples and a single repetition, provide relative expression of mRNA transcribed to cDNAs rather than absolute amounts. This limits the precision of the gene expression studies.

9. The study focuses on the downregulation of MMP2 and upregulation of fiber assembly proteins (elastin and LOX) particularly via the inhibition of MAPK pathway proteins (e.g., ERK, JNK, AKT etc.). Other pathways related to NO, such as the sGC-cGMP pathway, were not investigated, which represents a gap in pathway exploration.

10. The study exclusively explores Sodium Nitroprusside (SNP) as the NO donor. Exploring other NO donors such as GSNO, DETA/NO, SNAP etc. or combination therapies would offer a more comprehensive understanding of the strengths and limitations of different approaches and potential pro-matrix regenerative attributes or demerits of non-NO degradation drug byproducts.

11. The formulation of bLNPs with pre-incorprorated DSPE PEG-Biotin components presents challenges, including the need for excess lipopolymers. This renders the NP extrusion process challenging due to their viscosity and also causes significant volume leakage of the bLNP suspension. The pre-insertion technique modifies both the internal and external structures of bLNPs and this modification PEG-Biotin reduces available space for drug encapsulation within the core.

12. SNP release kinetics, relies on the quantification of nitrite at designated time points. Notably, both NO and nitrite have relatively short half-lives, ultimately oxidizing into nitrate. The quantification of SNP release in this study is based solely on the detection of nitrite at specific time points, offering only relative information on SNP release. Consequently, for a more precise evaluation of SNP release, it is essential to conduct comprehensive measurements of the absolute amounts of NO, nitrite, and nitrate.

13. The PCL and bPCL grafts exhibit autofluorescence, potentially masking fluorescence in other channels and leading to skewed results in imaging studies.

14. The decellularization step inadvertently causes some level of elastic matrix damage, introducing an undesirable element to the experimental design.

15. Acknowledging these limitations underscores the need for future research to address these gaps and refine the understanding of the proposed interventions.

5.3 Future Directions

Based on our findings in this study, I propose the following recommendations for future follow-up research:

1. Investigate the underlying mechanism governing the phenotypic switch of aHASMCs, with a specific focus on the NOTCH signaling pathway. Understanding the plasticity of aHASMCs through exploration of the NOTCH pathway could unveil potential therapeutic targets for treating AAAs.

2. Strengthen the validity of *in-vitro* assessments by incorporating cocultures of SMCs and macrophage phenotypes to mimic the crosstalk that occurs in a AAA tissue milieu. This approach aims to create a more clinically relevant AAA milieu, providing insights into the efficacy of SNPs as a drug for AAA treatment.

3. Explore a broader spectrum of NO donors or alternative options to assess their implications in maintaining AAA health. This exploration can contribute to a more comprehensive understanding of potential candidates for matrix regenerative therapy.

4. Broaden the scope of research by analyzing a diverse range of aHASMC samples obtained from various AAA donors. This approach will unveil patterns and responses that may vary among patients, paving the way for a personalized approach to AAA treatment.

5. Transition from static cultures to dynamic cultures simulates blood flow-induced stress on the aorta wall. This could be performed in a semi-high throughput manner in microfluidic device systems. This shift can offer a more in-depth analysis of both pathophysiology and potential therapeutic targets, providing valuable insights for AAA treatment.

6. Progress from simplified *in-vitro* models to *in-vivo* models that better mimic the dynamic conditions within living organisms. This transition is crucial for gaining a clearer understanding of the translational potential of SNP and SNP LCGs in treating AAAs.

7. Expand pathway exploration, especially those strongly linked to NO, such as sGC and cGMP pathways. Investigate their interactions with MAPKs, as well as their role in the transcriptional or translational regulation of elastin, LOX, and MMP expression. Additionally, explore lesser-known MAPK pathway proteins like mTOR or AKT to determine their relevance in AAAs.

8. Enhance the design of LNPs and LCGs to address challenges during preparation, including volume loss during extrusion and sterility issues. Aim for an encapsulation efficiency exceeding 80% to ensure a practical and effective drug delivery system.

9. Optimize the decellularization process to minimize matrix damage, ensuring that the resulting model accurately represents native tissue conditions. This refinement is crucial for improving the relevance and reliability of studies involving decellularized tissues.

10. Use of DNA assay for a quantitative evaluation of residual cells and precise determination of cell loss at each stage of the decellularization process, enhancing the accuracy of decellularization prediction.

11. Utilize recellularized dPCAs as xenografts in rats/mice aorta to establish an AAA model. This involves strategically placing the xenograft within the aorta, triggering an immune response marked by immune cell infiltration, antibody synthesis, and participation in ECM degradation, thereby facilitating aneurysm progression.

12. Evaluate the efficacy of LCGs in an *in-vivo* AAA rat or mice model to assess their performance in a more complex and dynamic physiological environment. This step is essential for determining the practical applicability of LCGs as a therapeutic intervention for AAAs.

13. Evaluate the practical efficacy of LCGs as a vascular stent or graft and explore their potential as a chargeable or rechargeable drug delivery system. This investigation seeks to reduce the necessity for high-risk surgeries by placing LCGs on the aorta's lumen and efficiently charging or recharging drug encapsulating nanocarriers onto the LCGs administered via tail vein injection with prior engineering and surface modification of LNPs (e.g., Biotin-Neutravidin).

List of References

1. Tsao CW, Aday AW, Almarzooq ZI, et al. Heart Disease and Stroke Statistics—2023 Update: A Report From the American Heart Association. Circulation 2023;147(8):e93–621.

2. Heart Disease Facts | cdc.gov [Internet]. Cent. Dis. Control Prev. 2023 [cited 2023 Jul 5];Available from: https://www.cdc.gov/heartdisease/facts.htm

3. Murray CJL. The Global Burden of Disease Study at 30 years. Nat Med 2022;28(10):2019–26.

4. Cardiovascular diseases [Internet]. [cited 2023 Jul 5];Available from: https://www.who.int/health-topics/cardiovascular-diseases

5. Droc I, Droc G, Buzila C, Calinescu FB. Abdominal Aortic Aneurysms (AAA) [Internet]. In: New Approaches to Aortic Diseases from Valve to Abdominal Bifurcation. Elsevier; 2018 [cited 2023 Sep 23]. p. 393–402.Available from: https://linkinghub.elsevier.com/retrieve/pii/B9780128099797000341

6. Abdominal Aortic Aneurysm | Society for Vascular Surgery [Internet]. [cited 2023 Sep 23];Available from: https://vascular.org/patients-and-referring-physicians/conditions/abdominal-aortic-aneurysm

7. Lo RC, Schermerhorn ML. Abdominal aortic aneurysms in women. J Vasc Surg 2016;63(3):839–44.

8. Lederle FA, Johnson GR, Wilson SE, et al. Prevalence and Associations of Abdominal Aortic Aneurysm Detected through Screening. Ann Intern Med 1997;126(6):441–9.

9. Li X, Zhao G, Zhang J, Duan Z, Xin S. Prevalence and Trends of the Abdominal Aortic Aneurysms Epidemic in General Population - A Meta-Analysis. PLoS ONE 2013;8(12):e81260.

10. Baxter BT, Terrin MC, Dalman RL. Medical Management of Small Abdominal Aortic Aneurysms. Circulation 2008;117(14):1883–9.

11. Kuivaniemi H, Ryer EJ, Elmore JR, Tromp G. Understanding the pathogenesis of abdominal aortic aneurysms. Expert Rev Cardiovasc Ther 2015;13(9):975–87.

12. Lu H, Du W, Ren L, et al. Vascular Smooth Muscle Cells in Aortic Aneurysm: From Genetics to Mechanisms. J Am Heart Assoc 2021;10(24):e023601.

13. Sivaraman B, Bashur CA, Ramamurthi A. Advances in biomimetic regeneration of elastic matrix structures. Drug Deliv Transl Res 2012;2(5):323–50.

14. Simmers P, Gishto A, Vyavahare N, Kothapalli CR. Nitric Oxide Stimulates Matrix Synthesis and Deposition by Adult Human Aortic Smooth Muscle Cells Within Three-Dimensional Cocultures. Tissue Eng Part A 2015;21(7–8):1455–70.

15. DiMusto PD, Lu G, Ghosh A, et al. Increased JNK in males compared to females in a rodent model of abdominal aortic aneurysm. J Surg Res 2012;176(2):687–95.

16. Ghosh A, DiMusto PD, Ehrlichman LK, et al. The Role of Extracellular Signal-Related Kinase During Abdominal Aortic Aneurysm Formation. J Am Coll Surg 2012;215(5):668-680.e1.

17. Aravani D, Foote K, Figg N, et al. Cytokine regulation of apoptosis-induced apoptosis and apoptosis-induced cell proliferation in vascular smooth muscle cells. Apoptosis 2020;25(9):648–62.

18. Sun J, Sukhova GK, Zhang J, et al. Cathepsin K deficiency reduces elastase perfusion-induced abdominal aortic aneurysms in mice. Arterioscler Thromb Vasc Biol 2012;32(1):15–23.

19. Sivaraman B, Ramamurthi A. Multifunctional Nanoparticles for Doxycycline Delivery Towards Localized Elastic Matrix Stabilization and Regenerative Repair. Acta Biomater 2013;9(5):6511–25.

20. Camardo A, Carney S, Ramamurthi A. Assessing the targeting and fate of cathepsin k antibody-modified nanoparticles in a rat abdominal aortic aneurysm model. Acta Biomater 2020;112:225–33.

21. Park H-S, Huh S-H, Kim M-S, Lee SH, Choi E-J. Nitric oxide negatively regulates c-Jun N-terminal kinase/stress-activated protein kinase by means of S-nitrosylation. Proc Natl Acad Sci U S A 2000;97(26):14382–7.

22. Zuckerbraun BS, Stoyanovsky DA, Sengupta R, et al. Nitric oxide-induced inhibition of smooth muscle cell proliferation involves S-nitrosation and inactivation of RhoA. 2007;292:9.

23. Okishima A, Koide H, Hoshino Y, et al. Design of Synthetic Polymer Nanoparticles Specifically Capturing Indole, a Small Toxic Molecule. Biomacromolecules 2019;20(4):1644–54.

24. Homayun B, Lin X, Choi H-J. Challenges and Recent Progress in Oral Drug Delivery Systems for Biopharmaceuticals. Pharmaceutics 2019;11(3):129.

25. Lou J, Duan H, Qin Q, et al. Advances in Oral Drug Delivery Systems: Challenges and Opportunities. Pharmaceutics 2023;15(2):484.

26. Jennewine B, Fox J, Ramamurthi A. Cathepsin K-targeted sub-micron particles for regenerative repair of vascular elastic matrix. Acta Biomater 2017;52:60–73.

27. Ruirui Z, He J, Xu X, et al. PLGA-based drug delivery system for combined therapy of cancer: research progress. Mater Res Express 2021;8(12):122002.

28. Akbarzadeh A, Rezaei-Sadabady R, Davaran S, et al. Liposome: classification, preparation, and applications. Nanoscale Res Lett 2013;8(1):102.

29. Liu P, Chen G, Zhang J. A Review of Liposomes as a Drug Delivery System: Current Status of Approved Products, Regulatory Environments, and Future Perspectives. Molecules 2022;27(4):1372.

30. Dwivedi R, Kumar S, Pandey R, et al. Polycaprolactone as biomaterial for bone scaffolds: Review of literature. J Oral Biol Craniofacial Res 2020;10(1):381–8.

31. Chow LW. Electrospinning Functionalized Polymers for Use as Tissue Engineering Scaffolds. Methods Mol Biol Clifton NJ 2018;1758:27–39.

32. Lindeman JHN, Abdul-Hussien H, van Bockel JH, Wolterbeek R, Kleemann R. Clinical Trial of Doxycycline for Matrix Metalloproteinase-9 Inhibition in Patients With an Abdominal Aneurysm: Doxycycline Selectively Depletes Aortic Wall Neutrophils and Cytotoxic T Cells. Circulation 2009;119(16):2209–16.

33. Matsumura JS, Chaikof EL. Continued expansion of aortic necks after endovascular repair of abdominal aortic aneurysms. J Vasc Surg 1998;28(3):422–31.

34. Li Y, Wang J, Gao Y, Zhu J, Wientjes MG, Au JL-S. Relationships between Liposome Properties, Cell Membrane Binding, Intracellular Processing, and Intracellular Bioavailability. AAPS J 2011;13(4):585–97.

35. Iyer AK, Khaled G, Fang J, Maeda H. Exploiting the enhanced permeability and retention effect for tumor targeting. Drug Discov Today 2006;11(17–18):812–8.

36. Circulatory System: Anatomy and Function [Internet]. Clevel. Clin. [cited 2023 Nov 4];Available from: https://my.clevelandclinic.org/health/body/21775-circulatory-system

37. Mathew P, Bordoni B. Embryology, Heart [Internet]. In: StatPearls. Treasure Island (FL): StatPearls Publishing; 2023 [cited 2023 Jul 2]. Available from: http://www.ncbi.nlm.nih.gov/books/NBK537313/

38. Tucker WD, Arora Y, Mahajan K. Anatomy, Blood Vessels [Internet]. In: StatPearls. Treasure Island (FL): StatPearls Publishing; 2023 [cited 2023 Jul 2]. Available from: http://www.ncbi.nlm.nih.gov/books/NBK470401/

39. Tinajero MG, Gotlieb AI. Recent Developments in Vascular Adventitial Pathobiology. Am J Pathol 2020;190(3):520–34.

40. Chronic Venous Insufficiency and Varicose Veins [Internet]. Dr Varshas Health Solut. 2021 [cited 2023 Nov 4];Available from: https://drvarsha.com/chronic-venous-insufficiency-and-varicose-veins/

41. Classification & Structure of Blood Vessels | SEER Training [Internet]. [cited 2023 Oct 25];Available from: https://training.seer.cancer.gov/anatomy/cardiovascular/blood/classification.html

42. Aorta: Anatomy and Function [Internet]. Clevel. Clin. [cited 2023 Jul 12];Available from: https://my.clevelandclinic.org/health/articles/17058-aorta-anatomy

43. Aorta anatomy - UF Health [Internet]. [cited 2023 Oct 25];Available from: https://ufhealth.org/conditions-and-treatments/aorta-anatomy

44. Wortmann M, Peters AS, Erhart P, Körfer D, Böckler D, Dihlmann S. Inflammasomes in the Pathophysiology of Aortic Disease. Cells 2021;10(9):2433.

45. Krüger-Genge A, Blocki A, Franke R-P, Jung F. Vascular Endothelial Cell Biology: An Update. Int J Mol Sci 2019;20(18):4411.

46. Liu VWT, Huang PL. Cardiovascular roles of nitric oxide: A review of insights from nitric oxide synthase gene disrupted mice†. Cardiovasc Res 2008;77(1):19–29.

47. Patel A, Fine B, Sandig M, Mequanint K. Elastin biosynthesis: The missing link in tissue-engineered blood vessels. Cardiovasc Res 2006;71(1):40–9.

48. Ozsvar J, Yang C, Cain SA, Baldock C, Tarakanova A, Weiss AS. Tropoelastin and Elastin Assembly. Front Bioeng Biotechnol 2021;9:643110.

49. Alexander MR, Owens GK. Epigenetic Control of Smooth Muscle Cell Differentiation and Phenotypic Switching in Vascular Development and Disease. Annu Rev Physiol 2012;74(1):13–40.

50. Stegemann JP, Hong H, Nerem RM. Mechanical, biochemical, and extracellular matrix effects on vascular smooth muscle cell phenotype. J Appl Physiol 2005;98(6):2321–7.

51. Structure and Function of Blood Vessels | Anatomy and Physiology II [Internet]. [cited 2023 Nov 4];Available from: https://courses.lumenlearning.com/suny-ap2/chapter/structure-and-function-of-blood-vessels/

52. Silver FH, Horváth I, Foran DJ. Viscoelasticity of the vessel wall: the role of collagen and elastic fibers. Crit Rev Biomed Eng 2001;29 3:279–301.

53. Cocciolone AJ, Hawes JZ, Staiculescu MC, Johnson EO, Murshed M, Wagenseil JE. Elastin, arterial mechanics, and cardiovascular disease. Am J Physiol Heart Circ Physiol 2018;315(2):H189–205.

54. Wenceslau CF, McCarthy CG, Earley S, et al. Guidelines for the measurement of vascular function and structure in isolated arteries and veins. Am J Physiol-Heart Circ Physiol 2021;321(1):H77–111.

55. Stenmark KR, Yeager ME, El Kasmi KC, et al. The Adventitia: Essential Regulator of Vascular Wall Structure and Function. Annu Rev Physiol 2013;75:23–47.

56. Mehta D, Malik AB. Signaling Mechanisms Regulating Endothelial Permeability. Physiol Rev 2006;86(1):279–367.

57. Garland CJ, Hiley CR, Dora KA. EDHF: spreading the influence of the endothelium. Br J Pharmacol 2011;164(3):839–52.

58. Lachaud CC, López-Beas J, Soria B, Hmadcha A. EGF-induced adipose tissue mesothelial cells undergo functional vascular smooth muscle differentiation. Cell Death Dis 2014;5(6):e1304.

59. Patel R, Cardneau JD, Colles SM, Graham LM. Synthetic smooth muscle cell phenotype is associated with increased nicotinamide adenine dinucleotide phosphate oxidase activity: Effect on collagen secretion. J Vasc Surg 2006;43(2):364–71.

60. Bacakova L, Travnickova M, Filova E, et al. The Role of Vascular Smooth Muscle Cells in the Physiology and Pathophysiology of Blood Vessels [Internet]. In: Sakuma K, editor. Muscle Cell and Tissue - Current Status of Research Field. InTech; 2018 [cited 2023 Oct 16]. Available from: http://www.intechopen.com/books/muscle-cell-and-tissue-current-status-of-research-field/the-role-of-vascular-smooth-muscle-cells-in-the-physiology-and-pathophysiology-of-blood-vessels

61. Shimizu K, Mitchell RN, Libby P. Inflammation and cellular immune responses in abdominal aortic aneurysms. Arterioscler Thromb Vasc Biol 2006;26(5):987–94.

62. Batra R, Suh MK, Carson JS, et al. IL-1β and TNF-α Impact Abdominal Aortic Aneurysm Formation by Differential Effects on Macrophage Polarization. Arterioscler Thromb Vasc Biol 2018;38(2):457–63.

63. Li Y, Takeshita K, Liu P-Y, et al. Smooth Muscle Notch1 Mediates Neointimal Formation After Vascular Injury. Circulation 2009;119(20):2686–92.

64. Beamish JA, He P, Kottke-Marchant K, Marchant RE. Molecular Regulation of Contractile Smooth Muscle Cell Phenotype: Implications for Vascular Tissue Engineering. Tissue Eng Part B Rev 2010;16(5):467–91.

65. Herity NA, Ward MR, Lo S, Yeung AC. Review: Clinical Aspects of Vascular Remodeling. J Cardiovasc Electrophysiol 1999;10(7):1016–24.

66. Baker AH, Zaltsman AB, George SJ, Newby AC. Divergent effects of tissue inhibitor of metalloproteinase-1, -2, or -3 overexpression on rat vascular smooth muscle cell

invasion, proliferation, and death in vitro. TIMP-3 promotes apoptosis. J Clin Invest 1998;101(6):1478–87.

67.   Dale MA, Ruhlman MK, Baxter BT. Inflammatory cell phenotypes in AAAs; their role and potential as targets for therapy. Arterioscler Thromb Vasc Biol 2015;35(8):1746–55.

68.   Desmoulière A, Chaponnier C, Gabbiani G. Tissue repair, contraction, and the myofibroblast. Wound Repair Regen Off Publ Wound Heal Soc Eur Tissue Repair Soc 2005;13(1):7–12.

69.   Gabbiani G. The myofibroblast in wound healing and fibrocontractive diseases. J Pathol 2003;200(4):500–3.

70.   Wolinsky H, Glagov S. A Lamellar Unit of Aortic Medial Structure and Function in Mammals. Circ Res 1967;20(1):99–111.

71.   Barallobre-Barreiro J, Loeys B, Mayr M, Rienks M, Verstraeten A, Kovacic JC. Extracellular Matrix in Vascular Disease, Part 2/4: JACC Focus Seminar. J Am Coll Cardiol 2020;75(17):2189–203.

72.   Kruegel J, Miosge N. Basement membrane components are key players in specialized extracellular matrices. Cell Mol Life Sci 2010;67(17):2879–95.

73.   Jana S, Hu M, Shen M, Kassiri Z. Extracellular matrix, regional heterogeneity of the aorta, and aortic aneurysm. Exp Mol Med [Internet] 2019 [cited 2023 Jul 13];51(12). Available from: https://www.ncbi.nlm.nih.gov/pmc/articles/PMC6923362/

74.   Yue B. Biology of the Extracellular Matrix: An Overview. J Glaucoma 2014;S20–3.

75.   Durbeej M. Laminins. Cell Tissue Res 2010;339(1):259–68.

76.   Hynes RO. Integrins: bidirectional, allosteric signaling machines. Cell 2002;110(6):673–87.

77.   Schwarzbauer JE, DeSimone DW. Fibronectins, Their Fibrillogenesis, and In Vivo Functions. Cold Spring Harb Perspect Biol 2011;3(7):a005041.

78.   Mosher D. Fibronectin. Elsevier; 2012.

79.   Wight TN. A Role for Proteoglycans in Vascular Disease. Matrix Biol J Int Soc Matrix Biol 2018;71–72:396–420.

80.   Halper J. Proteoglycans and diseases of soft tissues. Adv Exp Med Biol 2014;802:49–58.

81.   Spiro RG. Protein glycosylation: nature, distribution, enzymatic formation, and disease implications of glycopeptide bonds. Glycobiology 2002;12(4):43R-56R.

82.   Shriver Z, Raguram S, Sasisekharan R. Glycomics: a pathway to a class of new and improved therapeutics. Nat Rev Drug Discov 2004;3(10):863–73.

83.   Rienks M, Papageorgiou A-P, Frangogiannis NG, Heymans S. Myocardial Extracellular Matrix: An Ever-Changing and Diverse Entity. Circ Res 2014;114(5):872–88.

84.   Allahverdian S, Ortega C, Francis GA. Smooth Muscle Cell-Proteoglycan-Lipoprotein Interactions as Drivers of Atherosclerosis [Internet]. Berlin, Heidelberg: Springer Berlin Heidelberg; 2020 [cited 2023 Oct 19]. Available from: https://link.springer.com/10.1007/164_2020_364

85.   Humphrey JD. Possible Mechanical Roles of Glycosaminoglycans in Thoracic Aortic Dissection and Associations with Dysregulated TGF-β. J Vasc Res 2013;50(1):1–10.

86.   Paxton S, Peckham M, Knibbs A. The Leeds Histology Guide. 2003 [cited 2023 Aug 12];Available from: https://www.histology.leeds.ac.uk/tissue_types/connective/connective_groundS.php

87.   De Graffenried CL, Bertozzi CR. The roles of enzyme localisation and complex formation in glycan assembly within the Golgi apparatus. Curr Opin Cell Biol 2004;16(4):356–63.

88.   Menashi S, PoweR JT. Collagen in abdominal aortic aneurysm: Typing, content, and degradation. 1987;6(6):5.

89.   Shekhonin BV, Domogatsky SP, Muzykantov VR, Idelson GL, Rukosuev VS. Distribution of Type I, III, IV and V Collagen in Normal and Atherosclerotic Human Arterial Wall: Immunomorphological Characteristics. Coll Relat Res 1985;5(4):355–68.

90.   Cantini C, Kieffer P, Corman B, Limiñana P, Atkinson J, Lartaud-Idjouadiene I. Aminoguanidine and Aortic Wall Mechanics, Structure, and Composition in Aged Rats. Hypertension 2001;38(4):943–8.

91.   Belz GG. Elastic properties and Windkessel function of the human aorta. Cardiovasc Drugs Ther 1995;9(1):73–83.

92.   Karnik SK, Brooke BS, Bayes-Genis A, et al. A critical role for elastin signaling in vascular morphogenesis and disease. Development 2003;130(2):411–23.

93.   Debelle L, Tamburro AM. Elastin: molecular description and function. Int J Biochem Cell Biol 1999;31(2):261–72.

94.   Farrar DJ, Green HD, Bond MG, Wagner WD, Gobbeé RA. Aortic pulse wave velocity, elasticity, and composition in a nonhuman primate model of atherosclerosis. Circ Res 1978;43(1):52–62.

95.   Ma Z, Mao C, Jia Y, Fu Y, Kong W. Extracellular matrix dynamics in vascular remodeling. Am J Physiol - Cell Physiol 2020;319(3):C481–99.

96.   Ribeiro-Silva JC, Nolasco P, Krieger JE, Miyakawa AA. Dynamic Crosstalk between Vascular Smooth Muscle Cells and the Aged Extracellular Matrix. Int J Mol Sci 2021;22(18):10175.

97.   Humphrey JD, Tellides G. Central artery stiffness and thoracic aortopathy. Am J Physiol-Heart Circ Physiol 2019;316(1):H169–82.

98.   Shapiro SD, Endicott SK, Province MA, Pierce JA, Campbell EJ. Marked longevity of human lung parenchymal elastic fibers deduced from prevalence of D-aspartate and nuclear weapons-related radiocarbon. J Clin Invest 1991;87(5):1828–34.

99.   Halabi CM, Kozel BA. Vascular elastic fiber heterogeneity in health and disease. Curr Opin Hematol 2020;27(3):190–6.

100. Heinz A. Elastic fibers during aging and disease. Ageing Res Rev 2021;66:101255.

101. Hinek A, Rabinovitch M. 67-kD elastin-binding protein is a protective "companion" of extracellular insoluble elastin and intracellular tropoelastin. J Cell Biol 1994;126(2):563–74.

102. Hinek A, Mecham RP, Keeley F, Rabinovitch M. Impaired elastin fiber assembly related to reduced 67-kD elastin-binding protein in fetal lamb ductus arteriosus and in cultured aortic smooth muscle cells treated with chondroitin sulfate. J Clin Invest 1991;88(6):2083–94.

103. Schmelzer CEH, Heinz A, Troilo H, et al. Lysyl oxidase–like 2 (LOXL2)–mediated cross-linking of tropoelastin. FASEB J 2019;33(4):5468–81.

104. Hinderer S, Shena N, Ringuette L-J, et al. In vitro elastogenesis: instructing human vascular smooth muscle cells to generate an elastic fiber-containing extracellular matrix scaffold. Biomed Mater Bristol Engl 2015;10(3):034102.

105. Wagenseil JE. The matrix reloaded – Addressing structural integrity of the aortic wall in aneurysmal disease. Biomater Biosyst 2023;9:100072.

106. Canty EG, Kadler KE. Procollagen trafficking, processing and fibrillogenesis. J Cell Sci 2005;118(7):1341–53.

107. Collagen synthesis – MEHLMANMEDICAL [Internet]. 2023 [cited 2023 Aug 23];Available from: https://mehlmanmedical.com/collagen-synthesis/

108. Jaminon A, Reesink K, Kroon A, Schurgers L. The Role of Vascular Smooth Muscle Cells in Arterial Remodeling: Focus on Calcification-Related Processes. Int J Mol Sci 2019;20(22):5694.

109. Wang X, Khalil RA. Matrix Metalloproteinases, Vascular Remodeling, and Vascular Disease. Adv Pharmacol San Diego Calif 2018;81:241–330.

110. Visse R, Nagase H. Matrix metalloproteinases and tissue inhibitors of metalloproteinases: structure, function, and biochemistry. Circ Res 2003;92(8):827–39.

111. Corbel M, Boichot E, Lagente V. Role of gelatinases MMP-2 and MMP-9 in tissue remodeling following acute lung injury. Braz J Med Biol Res 2000;33(7):749–54.

112. Kandhwal M, Behl T, Singh S, et al. Role of matrix metalloproteinase in wound healing. Am J Transl Res 2022;14(7):4391–405.

113. Black RA, Rauch CT, Kozlosky CJ, et al. A metalloproteinase disintegrin that releases tumour-necrosis factor-alpha from cells. Nature 1997;385(6618):729–33.

114. Cheng XW, Huang Z, Kuzuya M, Okumura K, Murohara T. Cysteine Protease Cathepsins in Atherosclerosis-Based Vascular Disease and Its Complications. Hypertension 2011;58(6):978–86.

115. Murphy G. Tissue inhibitors of metalloproteinases. Genome Biol 2011;12(11):233.

116. Biljana E, Boris V, Cena D, Veleska-Stefkovska D. Matrix metalloproteinases (with accent to collagenases).

117. Jubaidi FF, Zainalabidin S, Taib IS, et al. The Role of PKC-MAPK Signalling Pathways in the Development of Hyperglycemia-Induced Cardiovascular Complications. Int J Mol Sci 2022;23(15):8582.

118. Chaikof EL, Dalman RL, Eskandari MK, et al. The Society for Vascular Surgery practice guidelines on the care of patients with an abdominal aortic aneurysm. J Vasc Surg 2018;67(1):2-77.e2.

119. Abdominal Aortic Aneurysm [Internet]. [cited 2023 Aug 19];Available from: http://healthlibrary.brighamandwomens.org/Search/85,P08247

120. Aggarwal S, Qamar A, Sharma V, Sharma A. Abdominal aortic aneurysm: A comprehensive review. Exp Clin Cardiol 2011;16(1):11–5.

121.	Nevitt MP, Ballard DJ, Hallett JW. Prognosis of abdominal aortic aneurysms. A population-based study. N Engl J Med 1989;321(15):1009–14.

122.	Lederle FA, Johnson GR, Wilson SE, et al. Rupture Rate of Large Abdominal Aortic Aneurysms in Patients Refusing or Unfit for Elective Repair. JAMA 2002;287(22):2968–72.

123.	Guirguis-Blake JM, Beil TL, Senger CA, Whitlock EP. Ultrasonography Screening for Abdominal Aortic Aneurysms: A Systematic Evidence Review for the U.S. Preventive Services Task Force. Ann Intern Med 2014;160(5):321–9.

124.	Kühnl A, Erk A, Trenner M, Salvermoser M, Schmid V, Eckstein H-H. Incidence, Treatment and Mortality in Patients with Abdominal Aortic Aneurysms. Dtsch Ärztebl Int 2017;114(22–23):391–8.

125.	Wise ES, Hocking KM, Brophy CM. Prediction of in-hospital mortality after ruptured abdominal aortic aneurysm repair using an artificial neural network. J Vasc Surg 2015;62(1):8–15.

126.	Katseni K, Chalkias A, Kotsis T, et al. The Effect of Perioperative Ischemia and Reperfusion on Multiorgan Dysfunction following Abdominal Aortic Aneurysm Repair. BioMed Res Int 2015;2015:598980.

127.	Kim HO, Yim NY, Kim JK, Kang YJ, Lee BC. Endovascular Aneurysm Repair for Abdominal Aortic Aneurysm: A Comprehensive Review. Korean J Radiol 2019;20(8):1247–65.

128.	Wanhainen A, Verzini F, Van Herzeele I, et al. Editor's Choice - European Society for Vascular Surgery (ESVS) 2019 Clinical Practice Guidelines on the Management of Abdominal Aorto-iliac Artery Aneurysms. Eur J Vasc Endovasc Surg Off J Eur Soc Vasc Surg 2019;57(1):8–93.

129.	Miyake T, Morishita R. Pharmacological treatment of abdominal aortic aneurysm. Cardiovasc Res 2009;83(3):436–43.

130.	Habashi JP, Judge DP, Holm TM, et al. Losartan, an AT1 antagonist, prevents aortic aneurysm in a mouse model of Marfan syndrome. Science 2006;312(5770):117–21.

131.	Camardo A, Seshadri D, Broekelmann T, Mecham R, Ramamurthi A. Multifunctional, JNK-inhibiting nanotherapeutics for augmented elastic matrix regenerative repair in aortic aneurysms. Drug Deliv Transl Res 2018;8(4):964–84.

132.	Nakahashi TK, Hoshina K, Tsao PS, et al. Flow Loading Induces Macrophage Antioxidative Gene Expression in Experimental Aneurysms. Arterioscler Thromb Vasc Biol 2002;22(12):2017–22.

133. Ailawadi G, Eliason JL, Roelofs KJ, et al. Gender Differences in Experimental Aortic Aneurysm Formation. Arterioscler Thromb Vasc Biol 2004;24(11):2116–22.

134. Parodi FE, Mao D, Ennis TL, Bartoli MA, Thompson RW. Suppression of experimental abdominal aortic aneurysms in mice by treatment with pyrrolidine dithiocarbamate, an antioxidant inhibitor of nuclear factor-kappaB. J Vasc Surg 2005;41(3):479–89.

135. Department of Medical and Health Sciences, Division of Drug Research, Linköping University, Sweden, Vorkapić E. Targeting vascular remodeling in abdominal aortic aneurysm : To identify novel treatment strategies and drug candidates [Internet]. Linköping University Electronic Press; 2016 [cited 2023 Nov 6]. Available from: http://urn.kb.se/resolve?urn=urn:nbn:se:liu:diva-127502

136. Peng H, Zhang S, Zhang Z, et al. Nitric oxide inhibits endothelial cell apoptosis by inhibiting cysteine-dependent SOD1 monomerization. FEBS Open Bio 2022;12(2):538–48.

137. Crawford CM, Hurtgen-Grace K, Talarico E, Marley J. Abdominal aortic aneurysm: an illustrated narrative review. J Manipulative Physiol Ther 2003;26(3):184–95.

138. Yoshimura K, Aoki H. Recent Advances in Pharmacotherapy Development for Abdominal Aortic Aneurysm. Int J Vasc Med 2012;2012:1–9.

139. Sun J, Sukhova GK, Yang M, et al. Mast cells modulate the pathogenesis of elastase-induced abdominal aortic aneurysms in mice. J Clin Invest 2007;117(11):3359–68.

140. Quintana RA, Taylor WR. Cellular Mechanisms of Aortic Aneurysm Formation. Circ Res 2019;124(4):607–18.

141. Lee E-J, Zheng M, Craft CM, Jeong S. Matrix metalloproteinase-9 (MMP-9) and tissue inhibitor of metalloproteinases 1 (TIMP-1) are localized in the nucleus of retinal Müller glial cells and modulated by cytokines and oxidative stress. PLOS ONE 2021;16(7):e0253915.

142. Davis FM, Rateri DL, Daugherty A. Mechanisms of aortic aneurysm formation: translating preclinical studies into clinical therapies. Heart 2014;100(19):1498–505.

143. Meghraoui-Kheddar A, Pierre A, Sellami M, Audonnet S, Lemaire F, Le Naour R. Elastin receptor (S-gal) occupancy by elastin peptides modulates T-cell response during murine emphysema. Am J Physiol-Lung Cell Mol Physiol 2017;313(3):L534–47.

144. Sagan A, Mrowiecki W, Mikolajczyk T, et al. Local inflammation is associated with aortic thrombus formation in abdominal aortic aneurysms. Relationship to clinical risk factors. Thromb Haemost 2012;108(5):812–23.

145. Rodgers JT. Vascular Endothelial Dysfunction and Effects on Arterial Wall Microstructure.

146. Su JB. Vascular endothelial dysfunction and pharmacological treatment. World J Cardiol 2015;7(11):719–41.

147. Tousoulis D, Kampoli A-M, Papageorgiou CTN, Stefanadis C. The Role of Nitric Oxide on Endothelial Function. :15.

148. Siwik DA, Colucci WS. Regulation of Matrix Metalloproteinases by Cytokines and Reactive Oxygen/Nitrogen Species in the Myocardium. Heart Fail Rev 2004;9(1):43–51.

149. Xiong W, Zhao Y, Prall A, Greiner TC, Baxter BT. Key roles of CD4+ T cells and IFN-gamma in the development of abdominal aortic aneurysms in a murine model. J Immunol Baltim Md 1950 2004;172(4):2607–12.

150. Murray PJ, Wynn TA. Protective and pathogenic functions of macrophage subsets. Nat Rev Immunol 2011;11(11):723–37.

151. Hata A, Chen Y-G. TGF-β Signaling from Receptors to Smads. Cold Spring Harb Perspect Biol 2016;8(9):a022061.

152. Hohmann S, Krantz M, Nordlander B. Yeast osmoregulation. Methods Enzymol 2007;428:29–45.

153. Maguire EM, Pearce SWA, Xiao R, Oo AY, Xiao Q. Matrix Metalloproteinase in Abdominal Aortic Aneurysm and Aortic Dissection. Pharmaceuticals 2019;12(3):118.

154. Johnson GL, Lapadat R. Mitogen-Activated Protein Kinase Pathways Mediated by ERK, JNK, and p38 Protein Kinases. Science 2002;298(5600):1911–2.

155. DiMusto PD, Lu G, Ghosh A, et al. Increased JNK in males compared to females in a rodent model of abdominal aortic aneurysm. J Surg Res 2012;176(2):687–95.

156. Laaksamo E, Tulamo R, Baumann M, et al. Involvement of Mitogen-Activated Protein Kinase Signaling in Growth and Rupture of Human Intracranial Aneurysms. Stroke 2008;39(3):886–92.

157. Yoshimura K, Aoki H, Ikeda Y, Furutani A, Hamano K, Matsuzaki M. Regression of Abdominal Aortic Aneurysm by Inhibition of c-Jun N-Terminal Kinase in Mice. Ann N Y Acad Sci 2006;1085.

158. Craige SM, Chen K, Blanton RM, Keaney JF, Kant S. JNK and cardiometabolic dysfunction. Biosci Rep 2019;39(7):BSR20190267.

159. Erk Signaling Pathway - Creative Diagnostics [Internet]. [cited 2023 Sep 12];Available from: https://www.creative-diagnostics.com/Erk-Signaling-Pathway.htm

160. Guo Y-J, Pan W-W, Liu S-B, Shen Z-F, Xu Y, Hu L-L. ERK/MAPK signalling pathway and tumorigenesis (Review). Exp Ther Med 2020;19(3):1997–2007.

161. The Nobel Prize in Physiology or Medicine 1998 [Internet]. NobelPrize.org. [cited 2023 Sep 2];Available from: https://www.nobelprize.org/prizes/medicine/1998/7543-the-nobel-prize-in-physiology-or-medicine-1998/

162. Loscalzo J, Welch G. Nitric oxide and its role in the cardiovascular system. Prog Cardiovasc Dis 1995;38(2):87–104.

163. Farah C, Michel LYM, Balligand J-L. Nitric oxide signalling in cardiovascular health and disease. Nat Rev Cardiol 2018;15(5):292–316.

164. Otsuka F, Finn AV, Yazdani SK, Nakano M, Kolodgie FD, Virmani R. The importance of the endothelium in atherothrombosis and coronary stenting. Nat Rev Cardiol 2012;9(8):439–53.

165. Pfeilschifter J, Eberhardt W, Huwiler A. Nitric oxide and mechanisms of redox signalling: matrix and matrix-metabolizing enzymes as prime nitric oxide targets. Eur J Pharmacol 2001;429(1):279–86.

166. Eberhardt W, Akool E-S, Rebhan J, et al. Inhibition of Cytokine-induced Matrix Metalloproteinase 9 Expression by Peroxisome Proliferator-activated Receptor α Agonists Is Indirect and Due to a NO-mediated Reduction of mRNA Stability. J Biol Chem 2002;277(36):33518–28.

167. Chen H, Wang DL. Nitric Oxide Inhibits Matrix Metalloproteinase-2 Expression via the Induction of Activating Transcription Factor 3 in Endothelial. 2003;

168. Akool E-S, Doller A, Müller R, et al. Nitric Oxide Induces TIMP-1 Expression by Activating the Transforming Growth Factor β-Smad Signaling Pathway *. J Biol Chem 2005;280(47):39403–16.

169. Park H-S, Huh S-H, Kim M-S, Lee SH, Choi E-J. Nitric oxide negatively regulates c-Jun N-terminal kinase/stress-activated protein kinase by means of S-nitrosylation. Proc Natl Acad Sci 2000;97(26):14382–7.

170. Eberhardt W, Pfeilschifter J. Nitric oxide and vascular remodeling: Spotlight on the kidney. Kidney Int 2007;72:S9–16.

171. Nichols SP, Storm WL, Koh A, Schoenfisch MH. Local delivery of nitric oxide: Targeted delivery of therapeutics to bone and connective tissues. Adv Drug Deliv Rev 2012;64(12):1177–88.

172. Cosby K, Partovi KS, Crawford JH, et al. Nitrite reduction to nitric oxide by deoxyhemoglobin vasodilates the human circulation. Nat Med 2003;9(12):1498–505.

173. Al-Sa'doni H, Ferro A. S-Nitrosothiols: a class of nitric oxide-donor drugs. Clin Sci Lond Engl 1979 2000;98(5):507–20.

174. Rose MJ, Mascharak PK. Fiat Lux: selective delivery of high flux of nitric oxide (NO) to biological targets using photoactive metal nitrosyls. Curr Opin Chem Biol 2008;12(2):238–44.

175. Grossi L, D'Angelo S. Sodium Nitroprusside: Mechanism of NO Release Mediated by Sulfhydryl-Containing Molecules. J Med Chem 2005;48(7):2622–6.

176. Zoupa E, Pitsikas N. The Nitric Oxide (NO) Donor Sodium Nitroprusside (SNP) and Its Potential for the Schizophrenia Therapy: Lights and Shadows. Molecules 2021;26(11):3196.

177. Ferrero R, Rodríguez-Pascual F, Miras-Portugal MT, Torres M. Comparative effects of several nitric oxide donors on intracellular cyclic GMP levels in bovine chromaffin cells: correlation with nitric oxide production. Br J Pharmacol 1999;127(3):779–87.

178. Homayun B, Lin X, Choi H-J. Challenges and Recent Progress in Oral Drug Delivery Systems for Biopharmaceuticals. Pharmaceutics 2019;11(3):129.

179. Patra JK, Das G, Fraceto LF, et al. Nano based drug delivery systems: recent developments and future prospects. J Nanobiotechnology 2018;16(1):71.

180. Afzal O, Altamimi ASA, Nadeem MS, et al. Nanoparticles in Drug Delivery: From History to Therapeutic Applications. Nanomaterials 2022;12(24):4494.

181. Richards DA, Maruani A, Chudasama V. Antibody fragments as nanoparticle targeting ligands: a step in the right direction. Chem Sci 2017;8(1):63–77.

182. Kulthe SS, Choudhari YM, Inamdar NN, Mourya V. Polymeric micelles: authoritative aspects for drug delivery. Des Monomers Polym 2012;15(5):465–521.

183. Fay F, Scott CJ. Antibody-targeted nanoparticles for cancer therapy. Immunotherapy 2011;3(3):381–94.

184. Dendrimers and their Applications as Novel Drug Delivery Carriers. J Appl Pharm Sci [Internet] 2013 [cited 2023 Nov 5];Available from: http://www.japsonline.com/abstract.php?article_id=1064

185. Sercombe L, Veerati T, Moheimani F, Wu SY, Sood AK, Hua S. Advances and Challenges of Liposome Assisted Drug Delivery. Front Pharmacol [Internet] 2015 [cited 2023 Nov 5];6. Available from: http://journal.frontiersin.org/article/10.3389/fphar.2015.00286

186. Zhang G, Sun J. Lipid in Chips: A Brief Review of Liposomes Formation by Microfluidics. Int J Nanomedicine 2021;Volume 16:7391–416.

187. Zhang H. Thin-Film Hydration Followed by Extrusion Method for Liposome Preparation [Internet]. In: D'Souza GGM, editor. Liposomes: Methods and Protocols. New York, NY: Springer New York; 2017. p. 17–22.Available from: https://doi.org/10.1007/978-1-4939-6591-5_2

188. Lombardo D, Kiselev MA. Methods of Liposomes Preparation: Formation and Control Factors of Versatile Nanocarriers for Biomedical and Nanomedicine Application. Pharmaceutics 2022;14(3):543.

189. Nsairat H, Khater D, Sayed U, Odeh F, Al Bawab A, Alshaer W. Liposomes: structure, composition, types, and clinical applications. Heliyon 2022;8(5):e09394.

190. Irby D, Du C, Li F. Lipid–Drug Conjugate for Enhancing Drug Delivery. Mol Pharm 2017;14(5):1325–38.

191. Bulbake U, Doppalapudi S, Kommineni N, Khan W. Liposomal Formulations in Clinical Use: An Updated Review. Pharmaceutics 2017;9(4):12.

192. Verma DD, Levchenko TS, Bernstein EA, Torchilin VP. ATP-loaded liposomes effectively protect mechanical functions of the myocardium from global ischemia in an isolated rat heart model. J Control Release Off J Control Release Soc 2005;108(2–3):460–71.

193. Ko YT, Hartner WC, Kale A, Torchilin VP. Gene delivery into ischemic myocardium by double-targeted lipoplexes with anti-myosin antibody and TAT peptide. Gene Ther 2009;16(1):52–9.

194. Lobatto ME, Fayad ZA, Silvera S, et al. Multimodal clinical imaging to longitudinally assess a nanomedical anti-inflammatory treatment in experimental atherosclerosis. Mol Pharm 2010;7(6):2020–9.

195. Camardo A, Seshadri D, Broekelmann T, Mecham R, Ramamurthi A. Multifunctional, JNK-inhibiting nanotherapeutics for augmented elastic matrix regenerative repair in aortic aneurysms. Drug Deliv Transl Res 2018;8(4):964–84.

196. Gacchina CE, Deb P, Barth JL, Ramamurthi A. Elastogenic Inductability of Smooth Muscle Cells from a Rat Model of Late Stage Abdominal Aortic Aneurysms. Tissue Eng Part A 2011;17(13–14):1699–711.

197. GeneCards - Human Genes | Gene Database | Gene Search [Internet]. [cited 2023 Nov 6];Available from: https://www.genecards.org/

198. Livak KJ, Schmittgen TD. Analysis of Relative Gene Expression Data Using Real-Time Quantitative PCR and the 2−ΔΔCT Method. Methods 2001;25(4):402–8.

199. Venkataraman L, Ramamurthi A. Induced Elastic Matrix Deposition Within Three-Dimensional Collagen Scaffolds. Tissue Eng Part A 2011;17(21–22):2879–89.

200. Swaminathan G, Stoilov I, Broekelmann T, Mecham R, Ramamurthi A. Phenotype-based selection of bone marrow mesenchymal stem cell-derived smooth muscle cells for elastic matrix regenerative repair in abdominal aortic aneurysms. J Tissue Eng Regen Med 2018;12(1):e60–70.

201. Labarca C, Paigen K. A simple, rapid, and sensitive DNA assay procedure. Anal Biochem 1980;102(2):344–52.

202. Stoilov I, Starcher BC, Mecham RP, Broekelmann TJ. Chapter 7 - Measurement of elastin, collagen, and total protein levels in tissues [Internet]. In: Mecham RP, editor. Methods in Cell Biology. Academic Press; 2018 [cited 2022 May 11]. p. 133–46.Available from: https://www.sciencedirect.com/science/article/pii/S0091679X17301292

203. Edwards CA, O'Brien WD. Modified assay for determination of hydroxyproline in a tissue hydrolyzate. Clin Chim Acta 1980;104(2):161–7.

204. Dudiki T, Mahajan G, Liu H, et al. Kindlin3 regulates biophysical properties and mechanics of membrane to cortex attachment. Cell Mol Life Sci 2021;78(8):4003–18.

205. Dahal S, Broekelman T, Mecham RP, Ramamurthi A. Maintaining Elastogenicity of Mesenchymal Stem Cell-Derived Smooth Muscle Cells in Two-Dimensional Culture. Tissue Eng Part A 2018;24(11–12):979–89.

206. Valverde M, Lozano-Salgado J, Fortini P, Rodriguez-Sastre MA, Rojas E, Dogliotti E. Hydrogen Peroxide-Induced DNA Damage and Repair through the Differentiation of Human Adipose-Derived Mesenchymal Stem Cells. Stem Cells Int 2018;2018:1615497.

207. Li K, Li Y, Mi J, Mao L, Han X, Zhao J. Resveratrol protects against sodium nitroprusside induced nucleus pulposus cell apoptosis by scavenging ROS. Int J Mol Med 2018;41(5):2485–92.

208. Rabkin SW, Klassen SS, Tsang MY. Sodium nitroprusside activates p38 mitogen activated protein kinase through a cGMP/PKG independent mechanism. Life Sci 2007;81(8):640–6.

209. Upchurch GR, Ford JW, Weiss SJ, et al. Nitric oxide inhibition increases matrix metalloproteinase–9 expression by rat aortic smooth muscle cells in vitro. J Vasc Surg 2001;34(1):76–83.

210. Souza-Pinto FJP, Moretti AIS, Cury V, Marcondes W, Velasco IT, Souza HP. Inducible nitric oxide synthase inhibition increases MMP-2 activity leading to imbalance between extracellular matrix deposition and degradation after polypropylene mesh implant. J Biomed Mater Res A 2013;101A(5):1379–87.

211. Kim K-H, Burkhart K, Chen P, et al. Tissue Inhibitor of Metalloproteinase-1 Deficiency Amplifies Acute Lung Injury in Bleomycin-Exposed Mice. Am J Respir Cell Mol Biol 2005;33(3):271–9.

212. Breynaert C, de Bruyn M, Arijs I, et al. Genetic Deletion of Tissue Inhibitor of Metalloproteinase-1/TIMP-1 Alters Inflammation and Attenuates Fibrosis in Dextran Sodium Sulphate-induced Murine Models of Colitis. J Crohns Colitis 2016;10(11):1336–50.

213. Phillips PG, Birnby LM. Nitric oxide modulates caveolin-1 and matrix metalloproteinase-9 expression and distribution at the endothelial cell/tumor cell interface. Am J Physiol-Lung Cell Mol Physiol 2004;286(5):L1055–65.

214. Eberhardt W, Beeg T, Beck K-F, et al. Nitric oxide modulates expression of matrix metalloproteinase-9 in rat mesangial cells. Kidney Int 2000;57(1):59–69.

215. Gacchina C, Brothers T, Ramamurthi A. Evaluating Smooth Muscle Cells from CaCl2-Induced Rat Aortal Expansions as a Surrogate Culture Model for Study of Elastogenic Induction of Human Aneurysmal Cells. Tissue Eng Part A 2011;17(15–16):1945–58.

216. Huang B, Zhao X, Zheng L-B, Zhang L, Ni B, Wang Y-W. Different expression of tissue inhibitor of metalloproteinase family members in rat dorsal root ganglia and their changes after peripheral nerve injury. Neuroscience 2011;193:421–8.

217. Hernandez-Barrantes S, Shimura Y, Soloway PD, Sang QA, Fridman R. Differential Roles of TIMP-4 and TIMP-2 in Pro-MMP-2 Activation by MT1-MMP. Biochem Biophys Res Commun 2001;281(1):126–30.

218. Cui X, Zhang J, Ma P, et al. cGMP-independent nitric oxide signaling and regulation of the cell cycle. BMC Genomics 2005;6:151.

219. Denninger JW, Marletta MA. Guanylate cyclase and the ·NO/cGMP signaling pathway. Biochim Biophys Acta BBA - Bioenerg 1999;1411(2):334–50.

220. Ridnour LA, Windhausen AN, Isenberg JS, et al. Nitric oxide regulates matrix metalloproteinase-9 activity by guanylyl-cyclase-dependent and -independent pathways. Proc Natl Acad Sci U S A 2007;104(43):16898–903.

221. Nguyen DHD, Hussaini IM, Gonias SL. Binding of Urokinase-type Plasminogen Activator to Its Receptor in MCF-7 Cells Activates Extracellular Signal-regulated Kinase 1 and 2 Which Is Required for Increased Cellular Motility. J Biol Chem 1998;273(14):8502–7.

222. Ghosh A, Lu G, Su G, et al. Phosphorylation of AKT and Abdominal Aortic Aneurysm Formation. Am J Pathol 2014;184(1):148–58.

223. Wang Z, Guo J, Han X, et al. Metformin represses the pathophysiology of AAA by suppressing the activation of PI3K/AKT/mTOR/autophagy pathway in ApoE−/− mice. Cell Biosci 2019;9(1):68.

224. Duda P, Akula SM, Abrams SL, et al. Targeting GSK3 and Associated Signaling Pathways Involved in Cancer. Cells 2020;9(5):1110.

225. Medunjanin S, Schleithoff L, Fiegehenn C, Weinert S, Zuschratter W, Braun-Dullaeus RC. GSK-3β controls NF-kappaB activity via IKKγ/NEMO. Sci Rep 2016;6:38553.

226. Salhi A, Farhadian JA, Giles KM, et al. RSK1 Activation Promotes Invasion in Nodular Melanoma. Am J Pathol 2015;185(3):704–16.

227. Cargnello M, Roux PP. Activation and Function of the MAPKs and Their Substrates, the MAPK-Activated Protein Kinases. Microbiol Mol Biol Rev MMBR 2011;75(1):50–83.

228. Ingram AJ, James L, Cai L, Thai K, Ly H, Scholey JW. NO Inhibits Stretch-induced MAPK Activity by Cytoskeletal Disruption. J Biol Chem 2000;275(51):40301–6.

229. Kim M-Y, Park J-H, Mo J-S, et al. Downregulation by lipopolysaccharide of Notch signaling, via nitric oxide. J Cell Sci 2008;121(9):1466–76.

230. Bedogni B, Warneke JA, Nickoloff BJ, Giaccia AJ, Powell MB. Notch1 is an effector of Akt and hypoxia in melanoma development. J Clin Invest 2008;118(11):3660–70.

231. Liu Z-J, Xiao M, Balint K, et al. Notch1 Signaling Promotes Primary Melanoma Progression by Activating Mitogen-Activated Protein Kinase/Phosphatidylinositol 3-Kinase-Akt Pathways and Up-regulating N-Cadherin Expression. Cancer Res 2006;66(8):4182–90.

232. Gurung R, Choong AM, Woo CC, Foo R, Sorokin V. Genetic and Epigenetic Mechanisms Underlying Vascular Smooth Muscle Cell Phenotypic Modulation in Abdominal Aortic Aneurysm. Int J Mol Sci 2020;21(17):6334.

233. Sorokin V, Vickneson K, Kofidis T, et al. Role of Vascular Smooth Muscle Cell Plasticity and Interactions in Vessel Wall Inflammation. Front Immunol [Internet] 2020 [cited 2022 May 9];11. Available from: https://www.frontiersin.org/article/10.3389/fimmu.2020.599415

234. Rensen SSM, Doevendans PAFM, van Eys GJJM. Regulation and characteristics of vascular smooth muscle cell phenotypic diversity. Neth Heart J 2007;15(3):100–8.

235. Zou L, Zhang J, Han J, et al. cGMP interacts with tropomyosin and downregulates actin-tropomyosin-myosin complex interaction. Respir Res 2018;19(1):201.

236. Shvetsova AA, Borzykh AA, Selivanova EK, Kiryukhina OO, Gaynullina DK, Tarasova OS. Intrauterine Nitric Oxide Deficiency Weakens Differentiation of Vascular Smooth Muscle in Newborn Rats. Int J Mol Sci 2021;22(15):8003.

237. Dai J, Sheetz MP. Membrane Tether Formation from Blebbing Cells. Biophys J 1999;77(6):3363–70.

238. Hong Z, Reeves KJ, Sun Z, Li Z, Brown NJ, Meininger GA. Vascular Smooth Muscle Cell Stiffness and Adhesion to Collagen I Modified by Vasoactive Agonists. PLOS ONE 2015;10(3):e0119533.

239. Farrell K, Simmers P, Mahajan G, et al. Alterations in phenotype and gene expression of adult human aneurysmal smooth muscle cells by exogenous nitric oxide. Exp Cell Res 2019;384(1):111589.

240. Abdul-Hussien H, Soekhoe RGV, Weber E, et al. Collagen Degradation in the Abdominal Aneurysm. Am J Pathol 2007;170(3):809–17.

241. Menashi S, PoweR JT. Collagen in abdominal aortic aneurysm: Typing, content, and degradation. 1987;6(6):5.

242. Hinderer S, Shen N, Ringuette L-J, et al. *In vitro* elastogenesis: instructing human vascular smooth muscle cells to generate an elastic fiber-containing extracellular matrix scaffold. Biomed Mater 2015;10(3):034102.

243. Wei S, Gao L, Wu C, Qin F, Yuan J. Role of the lysyl oxidase family in organ development (Review). Exp Ther Med 2020;20(1):163–72.

244. Sun H-J, Liu T-Y, Zhang F, et al. Salusin-β contributes to vascular remodeling associated with hypertension via promoting vascular smooth muscle cell proliferation and vascular fibrosis. Biochim Biophys Acta BBA - Mol Basis Dis 2015;1852(9):1709–18.

245. Abdul-Hussien H, Soekhoe RGV, Weber E, et al. Collagen Degradation in the Abdominal Aneurysm. Am J Pathol 2007;170(3):809–17.

246. Kolpakov V, Gordon D, Kulik TJ. Nitric Oxide–Generating Compounds Inhibit Total Protein and Collagen Synthesis in Cultured Vascular Smooth Muscle Cells. Circ Res 1995;76(2):305–9.

247. Mäki JM, Räsänen J, Tikkanen H, et al. Inactivation of the Lysyl Oxidase Gene Lox Leads to Aortic Aneurysms, Cardiovascular Dysfunction, and Perinatal Death in Mice. Circulation 2002;106(19):2503–9.

248. Finney J, Moon H-J, Ronnebaum T, Lantz M, Mure M. Human copper-dependent amine oxidases. Arch Biochem Biophys 2014;546:19–32.

249. Brophy CM, Tilson JE, Braverman IM, Tilson MD. Age of onset, pattern of distribution, and histology of aneurysm development in a genetically predisposed mouse model. J Vasc Surg 1988;8(1):45–8.

250. Umeda H, Aikawa M, Libby P. Liberation of Desmosine and Isodesmosine as Amino Acids from Insoluble Elastin by Elastolytic Proteases. Biochem Biophys Res Commun 2011;411(2):281–6.

251. Hedtke T, Schräder CU, Heinz A, et al. A comprehensive map of human elastin cross-linking during elastogenesis. FEBS J 2019;286(18):3594–610.

252. Horiguchi M, Inoue T, Ohbayashi T, et al. Fibulin-4 conducts proper elastogenesis via interaction with cross-linking enzyme lysyl oxidase. Proc Natl Acad Sci U S A 2009;106(45):19029–34.

253. Robb BW, Wachi H, Schaub T, Mecham RP, Davis EC. Characterization of an In Vitro Model of Elastic Fiber Assembly. Mol Biol Cell 1999;10(11):3595–605.

254. Du L, Rodgers J, Shazly T, Eberth JF, Lessner SM. THE EFFECT OF ENDOTHELIAL DYSFUNCTION ON AORTIC MECHANICS AND EXTRACELLULAR MATRIX MICROSTRUCTURE DURING AGE-RELATED VASCULAR REMODELING. :2.

255. Fitch RM, Vergona R, Sullivan ME, Wang Y-X. Nitric oxide synthase inhibition increases aortic stiffness measured by pulse wave velocity in rats. Cardiovasc Res 2001;51(2):351–8.

256. Nemcsik J, Kiss I, Tislér A. Arterial stiffness, vascular calcification and bone metabolism in chronic kidney disease. World J Nephrol 2012;1(1):25–34.

257. Blatter LA, Wier WG. Nitric oxide decreases [Ca2+]i in vascular smooth muscle by inhibition of the calcium current. Cell Calcium 1994;15(2):122–31.

258. Xu J, Shi G-P. Vascular wall extracellular matrix proteins and vascular diseases. Biochim Biophys Acta 2014;1842(11):2106–19.

259. Atkinson G, Bianco R, Di Gregoli K, Johnson JL. The contribution of matrix metalloproteinases and their inhibitors to the development, progression, and rupture of abdominal aortic aneurysms. Front Cardiovasc Med [Internet] 2023 [cited 2023 Oct 22];10. Available from: https://www.frontiersin.org/articles/10.3389/fcvm.2023.1248561

260. Bastola S, Kothapalli C, Ramamurthi A. Sodium Nitroprusside Stimulation of Elastic Matrix Regeneration by Aneurysmal Smooth Muscle Cells. Tissue Eng Part A [Internet] 2023 [cited 2023 Apr 3];Available from: https://doi.org/10.1089/ten.tea.2022.0169

261. Rigberg DA, Zingmond DS, McGory ML, et al. Age stratified, perioperative, and one-year mortality after abdominal aortic aneurysm repair: A statewide experience. J Vasc Surg 2006;43(2):224–9.

262. Greenhalgh RM. Prognosis of abdominal aortic aneurysm. BMJ 1990;301(6744):136.

263. Scott R a. P, Ashton HA, Kay DN. Abdominal aortic aneurysm in 4237 screened patients: Prevalence, development and management over 6 years. BJS Br J Surg 1991;78(9):1122–5.

264. Dahal S, Bastola S, Ramamurthi A. JNK2 silencing lipid nanoparticles for elastic matrix repair. J Biomed Mater Res A [Internet] [cited 2023 Oct 29];n/a(n/a). Available from: https://onlinelibrary.wiley.com/doi/abs/10.1002/jbm.a.37618

265. Wang Z, Zheng W, Wu Y, et al. Differences in performance of PCL-based vascular grafts as abdominal aorta substitutes in healthy and diabetic rats. Biomater Sci

266. Nosova AS, Koloskova OO, Nikonova AA, et al. Diversity of PEGylation methods of liposomes and their influence on RNA delivery. MedChemComm 2019;10(3):369–77.

267. Dokuchaeva AA, Mochalova AB, Timchenko TP, et al. In Vivo Evaluation of PCL Vascular Grafts Implanted in Rat Abdominal Aorta. Polymers 2022;14(16):3313.

268. Fukunishi T, Best CA, Sugiura T, et al. Tissue-Engineered Small Diameter Arterial Vascular Grafts from Cell-Free Nanofiber PCL/Chitosan Scaffolds in a Sheep Model. PLOS ONE 2016;11(7):e0158555.

269. Rasmussen MK, Pedersen JN, Marie R. Size and surface charge characterization of nanoparticles with a salt gradient. Nat Commun 2020;11(1):2337.

270. Costa P, Sousa Lobo JM. Modeling and comparison of dissolution profiles. Eur J Pharm Sci 2001;13(2):123–33.

271. Nguyen TX, Huang L, Liu L, Abdalla AME, Gauthier M, Yang G. Chitosan-coated nano-liposomes for the oral delivery of berberine hydrochloride. J Mater Chem B 2014;2(41):7149–59.

272. Gacchina C, Brothers T, Ramamurthi A. Evaluating Smooth Muscle Cells from CaCl2-Induced Rat Aortal Expansions as a Surrogate Culture Model for Study of Elastogenic Induction of Human Aneurysmal Cells. Tissue Eng Part A 2011;17(15–16):1945–58.

273. Camacho P, Fainor M, Seims KB, Tolbert JW, Chow LW. Fabricating spatially functionalized 3D-printed scaffolds for osteochondral tissue engineering. J Biol Methods 2021;8(1):e146.

274. Cai Z, Gu Y, Xiao Y, Wang C, Wang Z. Porcine carotid arteries decellularized with a suitable concentration combination of Triton X-100 and sodium dodecyl sulfate for tissue engineering vascular grafts. Cell Tissue Bank 2021;22(2):277–86.

275. Krajewski T. PROTEOLYZED VASCULAR EXTRACELLULAR MATRIX-COATED SUBSTRATES AS AN IN VITRO MODEL TO ASSESS ANEURYSMAL SMOOTH MUSCLE CELL BEHAVIOR.

276. Trooboff SW, Wanken ZJ, Gladders B, Columbo JA, Lurie JD, Goodney PP. Longitudinal Spending on Endovascular and Open Abdominal Aortic Aneurysm Repair. Circ Cardiovasc Qual Outcomes 2020;13(5):e006249.

277. Izzo C, Vitillo P, Di Pietro P, et al. The Role of Oxidative Stress in Cardiovascular Aging and Cardiovascular Diseases. Life 2021;11(1):60.

278. Thomas DD, Liu X, Kantrow SP, Lancaster JR. The biological lifetime of nitric oxide: Implications for the perivascular dynamics of NO and O2. Proc Natl Acad Sci U S A 2001;98(1):355–60.

279. Chen H, Ren X, Xu S, Zhang D, Han T. Optimization of Lipid Nanoformulations for Effective mRNA Delivery. Int J Nanomedicine 2022;Volume 17:2893–905.

280. Gjetting T, Arildsen NS, Christensen CL, et al. In vitro and in vivo effects of polyethylene glycol (PEG)-modified lipid in DOTAP/cholesterol-mediated gene transfection. Int J Nanomedicine 2010;5:371–83.

281. Wan J, Yang J, Lei W, et al. Anti-Oxidative, Anti-Apoptotic, and M2 Polarized DSPC Liposome Nanoparticles for Selective Treatment of Atherosclerosis. Int J Nanomedicine 2023;18:579–94.

282. Sut TN, Park H, Koo DJ, Yoon BK, Jackman JA. Distinct Binding Properties of Neutravidin and Streptavidin Proteins to Biotinylated Supported Lipid Bilayers: Implications for Sensor Functionalization. Sensors 2022;22(14):5185.

283. Vermette P, Gengenbach T, Divisekera U, Kambouris PA, Griesser HJ, Meagher L. Immobilization and surface characterization of NeutrAvidin biotin-binding protein on different hydrogel interlayers. J Colloid Interface Sci 2003;259(1):13–26.

284. Naseri H, Eskandari F, Jaafari MR, Khamesipour A, Abbasi A, Badiee A. PEGylation of cationic liposomes encapsulating soluble Leishmania antigens reduces the adjuvant efficacy of liposomes in murine model. Parasite Immunol 2017;39(11):e12492.

285. Reichert C, Borchard G. Noncovalent PEGylation, An Innovative Subchapter in the Field of Protein Modification. J Pharm Sci 2016;105(2):386–90.

286. Mansury D, Ghazvini K, Amel Jamehdar S, et al. Increasing Cellular Immune Response in Liposomal Formulations of DOTAP Encapsulated by Fusion Protein Hspx, PPE44, And Esxv, as a Potential Tuberculosis Vaccine Candidate. Rep Biochem Mol Biol 2019;7(2):156–66.

287. Jara-Quijada E, Pérez-Won M, Tabilo-Munizaga G, et al. Liposomes Loaded with Green Tea Polyphenols—Optimization, Characterization, and Release Kinetics Under Conventional Heating and Pulsed Electric Fields. Food Bioprocess Technol [Internet] 2023 [cited 2023 Nov 12];Available from: https://doi.org/10.1007/s11947-023-03136-8

288. Briuglia M-L, Rotella C, McFarlane A, Lamprou DA. Influence of cholesterol on liposome stability and on in vitro drug release. Drug Deliv Transl Res 2015;5(3):231–42.

289. Tang Q, Zhang W, Zhang C, et al. Oxymatrine loaded nitric oxide-releasing liposomes for the treatment of ulcerative colitis. Int J Pharm 2020;586:119617.

290. Miller MR, Megson IL. Recent developments in nitric oxide donor drugs. Br J Pharmacol 2007;151(3):305–21.

291. Papahadjopoulos D, Jacobson K, Nir S, Isac I. Phase transitions in phospholipid vesicles Fluorescence polarization and permeability measurements concerning the effect of temperature and cholesterol. Biochim Biophys Acta BBA - Biomembr 1973;311(3):330–48.

292. Wu IY, Bala S, Škalko-Basnet N, Di Cagno MP. Interpreting non-linear drug diffusion data: Utilizing Korsmeyer-Peppas model to study drug release from liposomes. Eur J Pharm Sci 2019;138:105026.

293. Bondonno CP, Liu AH, Croft KD, et al. Short-Term Effects of a High Nitrate Diet on Nitrate Metabolism in Healthy Individuals. Nutrients 2015;7(3):1906–15.

294. Hiller Y, Gershoni JM, Bayer EA, Wilchek M. Biotin binding to avidin. Oligosaccharide side chain not required for ligand association. Biochem J 1987;248(1):167–71.

295. Elia G. Biotinylation reagents for the study of cell surface proteins. Proteomics 2008;8(19):4012–24.

296. Kim M-C, Hong M-H, Lee B-H, Choi H-J, Ko Y-M, Lee Y-K. Bone Tissue Engineering by Using Calcium Phosphate Glass Scaffolds and the Avidin–Biotin Binding System. Ann Biomed Eng 2015;43(12):3004–14.

297. Gao J, Reibetanz U, Venkatraman S, Neu B. Biofunctionalization of Polyelectrolyte Microcapsules with Biotinylated Polyethylene Glycol-Grafted Liposomes. Macromol Biosci 2011;11(8):1079–87.

298. Pan J, Liu N, Shu L, Sun H. Application of avidin-biotin technology to improve cell adhesion on nanofibrous matrices. J Nanobiotechnology 2015;13(1):37.

299. Bhat VD, Truskey GA, Reichert WM. Fibronectin and avidin–biotin as a heterogeneous ligand system for enhanced endothelial cell adhesion. J Biomed Mater Res 1998;41(3):377–85.

300. Kuo SC, Lauffenburger DA. Relationship between receptor/ligand binding affinity and adhesion strength. Biophys J 1993;65(5):2191–200.

301. Chaurasiya P, Agarwal R, Loksh KR. Development and Characterization of Elastic Liposomes of Metronidazole for the Treatment of Bacterial Infection. J Drug Deliv Ther 2020;10(6-s):83–8.

302. Gurjar MV, DeLeon J, Sharma RV, Bhalla RC. Mechanism of inhibition of matrix metalloproteinase-9 induction by NO in vascular smooth muscle cells. J Appl Physiol 2001;91(3):1380–6.

303. Gurjar MV, Sharma RV, Bhalla RC. eNOS gene transfer inhibits smooth muscle cell migration and MMP-2 and MMP-9 activity. Arterioscler Thromb Vasc Biol 1999;19(12):2871–7.

304. Pustovrh MC, Jawerbaum A, White V, et al. The role of nitric oxide on matrix metalloproteinase 2 (MMP2) and MMP9 in placenta and fetus from diabetic rats. Reprod Camb Engl 2007;134(4):605–13.

305. Manabe S-I, Gu Z, Lipton SA. Activation of matrix metalloproteinase-9 via neuronal nitric oxide synthase contributes to NMDA-induced retinal ganglion cell death. Invest Ophthalmol Vis Sci 2005;46(12):4747–53.

306. Crapo PM, Gilbert TW, Badylak SF. An overview of tissue and whole organ decellularization processes. Biomaterials 2011;32(12):3233–43.

307. O'Neill JD, Anfang R, Anandappa A, et al. Decellularization of Human and Porcine Lung Tissues for Pulmonary Tissue Engineering. Ann Thorac Surg 2013;96(3):1046–56.

308. Dahan N, Zarbiv G, Sarig U, Karram T, Hoffman A, Machluf M. Porcine small diameter arterial extracellular matrix supports endothelium formation and media remodeling forming a promising vascular engineered biograft. Tissue Eng Part A 2012;18(3–4):411–22.

309. Kim H, Choi KH, Sung SC, Kim YS. Effect of ethanol washing on porcine pulmonary artery wall decellularization using sodium dodecyl sulfate. Artif Organs 2022;46(7):1281–93.

310. SMART - Servier Medical ART [Internet]. [cited 2023 Nov 22];Available from:

https://smart.servier.com/